LEO
& Friends

LEO
& Friends

The extraordinary dogs with the healing touch

Lyndsey Uglow

With Isabel George

With a foreword from James Middleton

HARPER element

HarperElement
An imprint of HarperCollins*Publishers*
1 London Bridge Street
London SE1 9GF

www.harpercollins.co.uk

HarperCollins*Publishers*
1st Floor, Watermarque Building, Ringsend Road
Dublin 4, Ireland

First published by HarperElement 2021

1 3 5 7 9 10 8 6 4 2

A catalogue record of this book is
available from the British Library

ISBN 978-0-00-846654-1

Printed and bound in the UK using 100%
renewable electricity at CPI Group (UK) Ltd

This book is produced from independently certified FSC™ paper
to ensure responsible forest management.

For more information visit: www.harpercollins.co.uk/green

About the Author

Kennel Club 'Friends for Life' 2020 winners Lyndsey and her therapy dog Leo represent everything there is to say about the powerful healing bond that exists between dogs and children.

Thanks to Lyndsey's pioneering work with therapy dogs, her team have helped more than 10,000 children, many critically ill, and their families at Southampton Children's Hospital; the healing value of Animal Assisted Intervention (AAI) is recognised by the Royal College of Nursing.

Wife, mother and daughter, Lyndsey has made this journey having endured and overcome her own mental health challenges and personal pain along the way.

Through the shadows of post-natal depression, loneliness in motherhood and the desperation of her young son's battle with Acute Myeloid Leukaemia, Lyndsey knows only too well the emotional rollercoaster experienced by parents, especially those supporting their children through critical illness and long hospital stays.

The healing bond with dogs that helped her, Lyndsey now shares with others – in the shape of a dynasty of exceptional golden retrievers. Including the incredible Leo – Lyndsey's hero on four paws.

For Mike, Harry and Ollie,
my family and friends, human and canine.
With thanks for your love and support.

Contents

Foreword

DOGS ... OUR HEALING COMPANIONS.

I love dogs.

As a self-confessed dog lover and admirer, it was an honour and a pleasure to present Lyndsey and Leo with the Kennel Club 'Friends for Life' winner's trophy in March 2020. I felt an immediate affinity with all that Lyndsey and her team are achieving in terms of Animal Assisted Intervention at Southampton Children's Hospital because to me, Leo and his canine friends represent all the good that can be found in the human-animal bond. All those patients' lives touched and enhanced by the presence of a dog – all that pure love and kindness on four legs.

On a personal level, I am pleased and proud to admit that my dogs have, in their own unique way, saved my life in my darkest hours. Ella, Zulu, Inka, Luna and Mabel are, I think, completely unaware of their gift to me but every day I want to tell them how deeply I appreciate the power of their unconditional love and companionship during my own battle with mental health and anxiety.

The warm light of kindness is present throughout this book and I can tell you right now that welcoming a dog into your life is like letting in sunshine; your world is immediately warmer and brighter. I say this because my appreciation of Animal Assisted Intervention came as I gradually realised any glimmers of light that I had encountered on my mental health journey came in the hours spent with my dogs. Somehow, I had been unable to find the right words to express my fears to my loving family, but my canine companions simply understood me – no words required.

I find it ironic that Winston Churchill named his depression the 'black dog' as it was my ever-faithful black spaniel, Ella, who showed me the way out of my darkness. Forever by my side, reading my emotions and body language, she accompanied me to all my therapy sessions and consistently distracted me from my sometimes crippling anxiety and feelings of isolation. I imagine that's how it must be for the children visited by Lyndsey and Leo – they feel an invisible connection through the dogs' silent understanding.

I'm not ashamed to say that in the beginning Ella probably knew me better than I knew myself and it was my therapeutic bond with her that led to my association with the charity Pets As Therapy (PAT). I can see now that Lyndsey and I had a similar journey discovering the charity and in both wanting our dogs to be PAT-assessed as soon as possible, so that we could go out and share that treasured canine love and support with others. Now, as a PAT Ambassador, I have the pleasure of seeing first-hand how a dog's company can be a massive support at the most challenging of times, including in hospitals, schools and care homes.

What Lyndsey started in 2012 as a Pets As Therapy volunteer has transcended into the Animal Assisted Intervention service that she and her team of volunteers now provide at Southampton Children's Hospital. Many of us will have a period of hospitalisation at some point in our lives and at that time everyone is likely to feel vulnerable. A visit from a therapy dog can ease those feelings.

In my experience dogs can be a powerful intervention in our lives, as the patients' stories in this book prove without a shadow of a doubt. The potential of the human-animal bond is, I think, there for us to explore and nurture and never take for granted. I, for one, will always be grateful for the dogs who have come into my life and helped me to understand, and who continue to walk beside me to support my mental recovery.

I believe that dogs teach us our worth in the love they give so freely and unconditionally. No wonder that, however long they are with us – for life, a visit, a moment at a hospital bedside – they leave behind a beautiful, indelible paw print on our heart.

James

James Middleton
PAT Ambassador and Mental Health Advocate

Prologue

I KNEW DOGS COULD MAKE A DIFFERENCE to the children's lives. I knew it the moment I watched a child, exhausted by pain and sickness, stretch out his hand to touch my dog's paw. And then … the smiles.

Every time I see that connection between a dog and a child in hospitals, in hospices and homes, I know that I'm privileged to be witnessing a little bit of canine magic.

One Sunday night …

> 'Lyndsey, can you bring in one of your dogs? There's a girl here in intensive care and we can't rouse her. She is eight years old and just had a resection of a brain tumour. She has no family or caregivers with her and we have successfully taken her off the ventilator but she's not even opened her eyes … she looks … sad. I wondered what we could do to help her as nothing seems to be working and I thought of the therapy dogs. We've talked to her about Leo and she has at least nodded. Can we tell her that you'll come in?'

'You were only with her fifteen minutes and Leo made her smile and speak! That was so powerful ... she trusted and felt safe with you and Leo, and now trusts us. Thank you. Leo achieved what we humans had failed ...'

(Donna Austin: Advanced Nurse Practitioner in Paediatric Intensive Care (PICU), Southampton Children's Hospital)

Part One:

Not all Superheroes Wear Capes!

1
Friends for Life

LEO WAS SNORING. Just looking at him reminded me why his nickname is 'Flump'. He is a fluffy lump, but to be fair, it had been a big day for all of us, especially Leo.

We were on the 125-mile drive back home to Hampshire when the wonderful reality dawned on me: it was true, we had won the Kennel Club 'Friends for Life' 2020 competition and although Leo was exhausted by his day in the limelight, he was happy. Spread out like a golden blanket, his two front paws curled over at the wrist, the left one trembling furiously. Maybe he was dreaming of digging on the beach or running from wheelie bins – he hates wheelie bins with a passion and cowers if he has to walk past one on the road!

We had shared an amazing day with the other four finalists in the competition, being ushered along to media photocalls, lined up for TV interviews and mobbed by hordes of dog-loving members of the public visiting *Crufts* – the world's biggest and greatest dog show.

On that Sunday, the fourth and final day of the show which is held annually at the National Exhibition Centre in Birmingham, we were treated like celebrities and Leo loved every second of being there as the winner of the category 'Child's Champion'. I couldn't help smiling at my amazing dog, leaning in to all the hugs that were on offer and giving Leo big hugs back.

Of course, I didn't make it easy – we took all of our team – six therapy dogs – with us! It was important to me that Leo was joined by his 'workmates' – Jessie, Quinn, Archie, Hattie and Milo. Thankfully, my fellow therapy dog handlers, Karen, Liz and Hannah, were there and my husband, Mike, 'volunteered' to lend a much-needed hand. I wanted our full canine line-up to share the 'Friends for Life' nomination, which had been submitted by the wonderful medical team at Southampton Children's Hospital. Win or lose, we were not going to let them down. This was our chance to show the world how therapy dogs can enhance lives, sometimes sadly to the end of life. That's why we had to be there in force – a cloud of retriever 'gold'. We were there for our brave young patients, for all those who were able to watch us in hospital or at home on TV, and those whose memory we hold close to our hearts.

Leo had received so many 'Good Luck' cards and messages from the children, some with lovely pictures of the dog himself: 'Go, Leo!', 'Leo's the best!', 'Leo ... my super-hero ...' The children amaze me every day and this time they surprised me because it's usually Leo wishing the children luck with their treatment and the patient receiving a 'Dogtor Leo' sticker or card. This was such a huge occasion and felt like a massive responsibility. We could not let them down.

So, there we were in the cavernous *Crufts* main arena with the other finalists, all new-found friends, and all of us standing nervously in the glare of the spotlights, a capacity crowd clapping and cheering, Channel 4 TV cameras hovering to capture the moment the winner stepped forward to lift the impressive glass trophy. I felt a flurry of butterflies in my tummy and at the same time a wave of calm coming up through the lead from Leo, who was sitting at my feet, keeping me anchored just when I needed it most.

Then, waiting on the edge of the longest pause ... I heard it, riding over the noise of the now hushed and expectant crowd – 'Friends for Life' Ambassador James Middleton's voice: 'And the winner is ... Lyndsey and Leo!'

It was an extraordinary moment. Even though I had convinced myself one of the others would win, it was wonderful to hear those words. I felt like I was smiling from the inside.

A wave of applause swelled up and high around the auditorium but I couldn't see faces, only the bright spotlights, like flashing stars. My eyes tried to follow each one as they bounced around in all directions and my thoughts turned to our 'angel patients', the ones who'd had Leo's comfort in their last days or hours, and how they would have loved celebrating with us. One of those little angels was Zoé ...

When we first met, the thing I noticed straight away about Zoé was her beautiful red painted toe and fingernails. She loved being pampered, she loved ladybirds and she loved Leo.

When we saw her for the last time, the monster, inoperable DIPG (diffuse intrinsic pontine glioma) brain tumour had her firmly and finally in its grasp, closing down her body in its wicked way. Leo knew his way around Naomi House children's hospice and swaggered towards Zoé's bed, where I placed him close to her outstretched hand.

Her eyesight was failing but although she couldn't see him clearly her smiles were a signal that she could feel Leo's warmth and softness as her little fingers slowly ruffled through his coat. Leo sniffed her fingers and painted toes as he had done many times before ... she could feel the tickle of his breath, which made her so happy and smiley. For one incredibly special moment, Zoé's parents and grandparents shared some time stroking Leo, too. He seemed to calmly know why and how much to give of himself to each person at that moment in that room. Photographs were taken with Leo to capture the smiles. Hugs were given and received before we left.

Zoé was just eight years old. She loved dogs ... especially Leo.

2
Leo's courage lies deeper

WHENEVER I LOOK AT LEO I see all the wonderful qualities of a golden retriever: he is, like his friends, intelligent, friendly, trustworthy, loyal and kind, and then there's something that I call an extra-special ingredient in Leo's personality. I recognised it in an urban dictionary description of someone named Leo: '... a person who makes you feel comfortable and secure about yourself ... genuinely the sweetest person ever.'

If Leo were a person, he'd be one of the good guys – in the words of Catherine, his breeder: 'You don't often get a goody-two-shoes like him!' Leo is his own dog, so completely dappy, gentle and kind, and that's why I believe that I found him the role he was meant for in life. It was on the advice of a friend from the Southern Golden Retriever Society, who advised me: 'The thing about the dog world is you must do your own thing. Do what interests you and what your dog enjoys.' And, together, that's exactly what we have done.

And when we are together, he is always as close as he can get and even on walks, he makes sure that he stays in my eyeline just so that he can dash in for any fuss or games that may be on offer.

Leo, is, physically, head to paw, a typically regal golden retriever, but he's not the outdoor, field dog type. He will run out with the grace of a show dog to look at the birds flying around but as for locating and retrieving one of them in his mouth – he is no more likely to do that than I am! He also hates walking on rainy days and, given the choice, he'd spend every day lying on a sofa accepting love and affection.

Being a member of a multi-dog household has probably saved Leo from the full-time role of adored couch potato and exposed his more active talent – his natural empathy for people. Leo nudges the needy, he leans into them to offer comfort. And that, I think, is what makes him my ideal healthcare partner.

My Leo, or to give him his full KC (Kennel Club) registered title: Rayleas Grand Master Leo at Solentgold, is, despite his name and golden coat, no Lion King. But when he's carrying out his duties there is no doubt at all that he thinks he is king of the corridors at Southampton Children's Hospital (SCH). In his world, that special environment, he is in every way the perfect mild-mannered therapy dog. Ironically, it's the only place where he also shows his stubborn streak: at times when he feels he needs to stay with a patient or that he's missed someone on his rounds, he puts the brakes on and I have to take him back until he is happy that his job is done. Maybe that's where the working part of him comes through and the bit I can relate to most of all: his commitment to his work is instinctive, total and knows no bounds. It's that 'If a job's worth doing, it's worth doing well' approach that I admire in Leo. He just has 'it' and, who knows, maybe without Leo, I would never have found my true way in this world either.

To be honest, Leo isn't the bravest of dogs but he is very handsome. He qualified for *Crufts* in the showring but, ultimately, he didn't like the look of the bigger dogs and, typically, he sidesteps any confrontation. It's not an environment Leo enjoys, which is probably down to the fact I am not a particularly confident handler in competition. Instead, he prefers to be his kind, empathic self, where these qualities are most valued – with the children on the wards. And when he's not playing, running, or working, he's happy sleeping and snuggling.

You see, Leo's kind of courage lies in a deep place, right alongside the huge dollops of calm and peace that dominate his character. When I watch him approach people we visit, it's always with care, never boisterous, or pushy. He sidles up and just puts himself within easy reach. He loves working in the hospital, meeting the children; it's where he's so relaxed doing what he does best, always aware that I am there to position him if he throws me that special look that says he wants to be closer to help someone. Somehow, he always gets it right.

I secretly hoped that this dream of the Kennel Club 'Friends for Life' win would come true – for the team and every child and parent who knows what it feels like to experience that touch … a touch that can only come from a therapy dog, so very often a golden light in the darkness.

On that special Sunday I was amazed by the number of people who came up to Leo and knelt down to hug him and whisper 'thank you' in his ear. People were chatting to all of us on the team and saying that they or a relative had experienced one of our visits. It was amazing to me how far around the country, experience of our volunteering had spread. I thought of the 10,000+ lives touched by the team since we started this journey in 2012, so many smiles in the shadow of trauma, critical and terminal illness, grief and loss. All thanks to the power of Animal Assisted Intervention reaching out in a way that, at one time not so long ago, I could only imagine was even remotely possible.

Standing there with Leo, his tail gently sweeping from side to side, his eager paws treading the green carpet, it hit me how long and often painful the journey had been to reach this very special moment. I felt the tears spiking their way to the surface, but it wasn't their turn, not today. This wasn't my day; it belonged to Leo and the others and, this time, it was my turn to be brave for them. At least that's what I thought until I saw my dog looking to me as if to say: 'This is fun, boss, so, tell me ... what's next?'

In the whirl of it all I remember being presented with the wonderful trophy and being asked to share a few words about our win with the audience and the television viewers, which was easy to do with Leo there for support. I could see my teammates in the wings, full of emotion and joy, and Mike had the biggest beam of pride on his face.

Leo's special kind of bravery made me brave on that special day at *Crufts* – that's the kind of superhero he is, every day, without even knowing it. On that big day for us, my handsome, faithful, intuitive and extraordinarily special golden retriever was where he is so very often – right by my side, simply doing what he does best, being himself ... just being a dog.

He took the applause in his usual laid-back, cool-guy way and all the fuss that was coming in his direction too. It was then I noticed the man and woman standing next to me, smiling through their tears: Alice's parents were there to support us. Alice Razza ... beautiful and brave Alice (who you will hear more of later). She loved her canine cuddles and the first time it happened her mother cried with happiness.

Seeing Alice's parents, Debbie and Rik, stand with us that day was a moment that snatched a heartbeat to remind me why we go into the hospital with our dogs. And how on earth I got into all of this amazing work that has simply, sometimes achingly, taken over my life.

I am just the dog handler but I carry these stories, and all our angel patients, in my head and in my heart and I know that I always will. And that's why I need to feel at my strongest before I allow myself to recall how this incredible journey with Leo and his friends began.

3

Fighting the dark thoughts

I REMEMBER SOMEONE SAYING TO ME: 'What on earth have you got to be down about?'

Believe me, back at the end of 2000 I asked myself the same question a million times over. There I was, seven years married to a wonderful, loving man, two beautiful young sons and a home in a Hampshire village. People were right, what on earth could I possibly be down about?

I was needed by everyone around me: my young boys, Harry and Ollie, and Mike, my orthopaedic surgeon husband, they all relied on me and I liked that. I'm proud to say that my life purpose, as wife and mother, has always made me feel hugely privileged. I know that my existence has always been valuable to them and each role has defined me as a useful person, and if there's one thing I need to be, it's a useful person. At the turn of the millennium, we were in a busy place with little or no time to question anything as there was too much to get done and I was happy to be needed. In the summer of 2000, we had returned from living in Sydney, a fabulous time for all of us, while Mike was working there, and in some ways, it was a pity we had to come home. But our demons live in our heads, not our suitcases, and my demons seemed determined to make their presence felt.

On the outside I wore my happy face but, in truth and in the shadows, happiness kept eluding me. I wanted it but somehow I couldn't grasp it and bring it close to me. Underneath all the layers of others' needs – who was the real Lyndsey? Where on earth had she gone? Had she been left behind in Sydney?

I could have shown my vulnerability, talked to someone and maybe exorcised those demons, but I felt there wasn't the time or space in my world to wallow in my own emotions or risk anything new, so I decided to stick with my tried-and-tested coping mechanism of routine. I had spent years honing my 'safe' behaviour patterns to cope, to survive; I knew them and as long as I was able to hold them tight, they kept me safe.

So, I kept my new mum emptiness exactly where I could control it ... on the inside. As the dark grey clouds of overwhelm and confusion swirled around me, I found a smile so no one would see my pain, or worse still, judge me for it. I put myself on 'smart-mum autopilot' and kept all my plates spinning crazily because the alternative was too scary to contemplate. If I stopped, everything would crash to the ground and then what would happen?

Who would I be then?

There was a dark void inside me. I could feel it. But reaching for help would only make everything worse and betray everyone who loved me, the last people on earth that I wanted to hurt. For a while I felt that my grip on the emotional aspects of my life was fragile.

Dark thoughts come in shades and lurk in the shadows of the day and night, and years later, thinking back over my volunteering journey, I remember one of our teenage patients, Becky, who knew all about dark places but whose love for Leo, she says, saved her life.

When I first saw Becky, she was lying bruised and battered in a bed on Southampton Children's Hospital G3 trauma and orthopaedic ward. The clinical staff told me that Becky's parents had seen me with Leo on the ward and wondered if I would drop by their daughter's bed next time I was in to say hello as she loved dogs and it just might lift her spirits. It was an invitation I was happy to accept; I just hoped that Leo and I could bring something to Becky as her injuries were so severe and she must have been in excruciating pain. I learned that this brave 16-year-old's fight for life in a hospital bed had begun with a two-year battle with depression, anxiety and anorexia nervosa. Withdrawing from friends and family, pushing away anyone who tried to help her, she reached a point where, as she later told me herself: 'I had no urge to carry on fighting my own mind on a daily basis ... and so I made the decision to end my life.' At breaking point, on 21 May 2014, Becky climbed to the top of a five-storey car park and jumped.

The girl I saw lying there had broken and missing teeth, internal and external stitches in her jaw, a cast on her left arm up to above her elbow and heavy plaster casts on each leg, with a wound drain in her right foot. Until then all the outside world had seen was a clever and completely independent teenager who was working towards her GCSEs and now she was not even able to turn herself in bed. I imagined that she must be terrified and terribly lonely, but I knew for sure that I was in the presence of an extraordinary survivor.

The lovely staff on G3 were pleased to see us and greeted Leo with the usual smiles and fuss, which, of course, he loved. I saw Becky's parents and they smiled when they caught sight of Leo plodding along at my side, his golden head held high and his eyes focused on what I'm sure he sees as his 'hospital rounds'. We are always aware that not everyone welcomes a four-legged visitor or is well enough to accommodate a dog's presence when they are surrounded by an array of hospital equipment, but, in Becky's case, there was every reason to believe that our visit would be a dose of the best kind of medicine. I had been told that she didn't believe her parents when they told her that they had seen a dog visiting on the ward, so I guessed that Leo would be a bit of a surprise!

It was almost as if Leo knew that he was going to be making this extra visit because he naturally led the way across the bay to the bed where Becky was lying. I swear my dog has a sixth sense – as we approached, he started to put in a bit of a prance rather than his usual plod until he was close to Becky's bedside, his brown eyes shining and his head turning backwards and forwards, looking from me to Becky, his canine body language telling me clearly that he wanted to get closer to our patient. I looked at

Becky and saw her eyes light up as she attempted a smile, even though she had a broken jaw; just the glint in her eyes was absolutely priceless. At least now she knew that her parents were telling the truth – there really was a lady with a dog in the hospital!

Becky's bed had already been prepared with an incontinence protection pad spread out ready for Leo's front paws to rest on. He looked so handsome after his usual wash-and-brush-up, his hair dried and groomed for his visit. I supported his body and raised his front paws to be beside Becky so she felt him close to her, his paws there to touch when she was ready. It was only a few seconds before Becky's hand found Leo's paw and there was the connection and the smiles for me and Becky's parents to see. She stroked his chest fur, running her fingers through his thick coat over and over, and Leo smiled his appreciation for all the fuss and attention. Whatever was said between them was done without words and for that short time, Becky said that the pain left her body and her bones didn't seem to be broken. She told me how, for just those moments, she was 'a normal teenager again, having fun with a dog.'

It was a great visit, by that I mean it had all the essential ingredients for Leo's 'intervention' to be a therapeutic support to Becky: the calm connection that just happened in the moment of touch and mirrored smiles. I knew that it was the start of another relationship that was bound to cut into my heart. I saw a vulnerable teenager lying there and I saw a part of my younger self – not in her physical pain but in the emotional challenge and confusion of teen pressures that brought her to that place, to the top of that multi-storey car park. Who would have imagined that a golden retriever called Leo would be her superhero? He is, after all, the dog my sons occasionally call Scooby-Doo, Snoozy boy or, at his least alert, Eeyore!

That visit took place in the same week that Becky's parents received some bad news about the prognosis of her right foot, which was still in pieces and with amputation looking like the only way ahead. The complex fracture in her left foot had been fixed with pins and screws but her right foot was a smashed mess and so painful that morphine wasn't touching it. I heard that she had screamed for hours and couldn't bear anyone or anything to touch or even be near her foot and especially her toes, not even a bed sheet. She had a condition called dysaesthesia, which meant any touch felt abnormal and really unpleasant. To help, one of the physiotherapists had taken to writing 'DO NOT TOUCH MY TOES' on Becky's plaster cast.

It was uncertain how many of the nerves in her right foot were intact, which made amputation seem all the more possible. I couldn't help thinking of how this young girl's life had changed in seconds and her parents were powerless to help her as she faced the new mental turmoil of accepting life as a potential amputee. Mike, as Becky's consultant, had a word with me about the visits and the difference the first one with Leo had made to her psychologically. Just laying eyes on Leo had made her smile for the first time since she arrived on the ward. And then the big ask ... How soon could I see Becky again?

It had to be soon.

In many ways the afternoon of the next visit was just like any other, except that I knew, whatever happened, we had to see Becky on our rounds. When we walked into G3, I saw Becky in her wheelchair as her dad was about to wheel her off the ward for a change of scenery, so we stopped for a chat. Becky asked if she could give Leo a treat and that, of course, came with lots of strokes and squishy Leo cuddles. It was lovely to see Becky smiling and when she asked if she could have a photo taken with Leo, I was only too happy to position him by her side. He is exceptionally good at being 'positioned', which is why I sometimes call him my Playdough! But what happened next left me totally speechless. After sitting handsomely for his moment on camera, Leo immediately turned his attention to his patient's blue and swollen toes: first giving her right foot a really good sniff all around the bottom of the cast, and then, quick as a flash, he licked the previously unbearably painful, untouchable and, by now, very smelly toes poking out of the plaster cast.

I don't think any of us could believe it: Becky actually felt Leo gently licking her toes! Seeing that fluffy golden retriever snuffling around her feet was a surreal but heart-stopping moment for everyone in the room. For Becky, it was a sign of hope that her foot was going to be OK. It was a turning point for her worried parents, not to mention Mike as her surgeon and the whole clinical team who really feared that the nerves were too badly damaged for the foot to survive. I'm not sure if we were all laughing or crying that day. Instead of getting told: 'Leo, no licking!' my dappy dog was the hero of the moment and quite rightly enjoyed all the excitement and the extra fuss and cuddles. He had no idea what he had just done for Becky and her family.

We saw Becky many times during her three-month stay on G3 ward. All visits just as lovely as the one before and all involving cuddles, strokes and feeding Leo the occasional treat. Becky told me that it wasn't long after meeting Leo that she decided that she wanted a golden retriever as her 'recovery puppy'. I took that as a real compliment and I know Leo would have if he'd understood what was really going on. But who knows ... maybe he did?

There's no doubt about it, that toe-licking victory moment was amazing, although as a therapy dog handler I have to admit to feeling a pang of shame – therapy dogs are not meant to lick at all. In Leo's defence, and in defence of all dogs who can't resist investigating smelly things, they were probably the smelliest toes on the planet, as no one had been able to get near enough to give them even a cursory clean. Leo just couldn't resist!

Over the weeks, we watched Becky gradually regain her strength and discover an incredibly unyielding determination to recover. She wanted to go home to her loving family and, perhaps more than anything, prepare to welcome her puppy. After Becky was discharged, we kept in touch and Leo went to see her at home, which was such a special time; it was just wonderful to see that ongoing connection between them. I saw how they shared a special 'space', just the two of them, which I can only imagine was formed in those early visits when the days in hospital were so long and so painful for Becky. It was also a relationship that, unusually, blossomed from the moment Leo licked Becky's toes!

Later, Becky wrote to me:

> I don't think I would be where I am now if Leo had not been with me that day. I began to believe that I could work hard and keep my foot and my family believed it too and they motivated me to stay strong ... In a way Leo was my first dog. He taught me all about the love that dogs provide; they don't care what weight you are or what you ate that day, they don't care if you're depressed or anxious ... they just love you unconditionally. Leo was all of that to me, and then when Mum and Dad promised me that when I was physically recovered and home I could have a puppy of my own, I had that to look forward to. I am fortunate enough to have my puppy, Monty, but it was Leo who saved me.

Becky sharing her thoughts on Leo with me really indicated the level of connection they had and that really affected me. It happened again when we all appeared together in an episode of Channel 4's *Supervet in the Field* with Noel Fitzpatrick. Becky told the Supervet all about her journey and how Leo had helped her through all the stages of her recovery, when her body was broken, bruised and contorted with pain and she was afraid of the future. And he did it by just being present, by being himself and accepting her just as she was every time he saw her. I had to laugh when she mentioned the time Leo popped into one of her clinic appointments, wearing his dress-up lion's mane wig! It seemed both amazing and surreal for Leo and I to be sitting there on the television with Becky telling her story. I was so proud of them both: Becky for winning her fight to survive and Leo for being such a valued 'person' in her recovery.

And no one could imagine my pride and inner glow the next time I saw Becky, on Southampton's paediatric intensive care unit (PICU). This time she wasn't there as a patient but as a second-year nursing degree student. Inspired by the nurses who cared for her on G3, Becky set her sights on graduating as one, determined to provide other families and children with the same high level of care that she had received when she needed it most.

I admire Becky, her strength and resilience as a teenager finding her way through, fighting her shadows with the amazing support of her mum, dad and sister as well as her loyal friends from university and ice-skating (yes, she is an ice-skating champion too). Becky was not alone on her journey and it was, as it always is, a privilege to play our part too. Leo, even if he could talk, would never betray a single secret Becky shared with him during those visits. He listened, never judged and made sure that he was beside her for as long as she needed him.

The privilege of having someone else to distract you from your own stresses is very powerful and at times, when I've had troubles in my life, it has been the dogs and the therapy visits that have been the most pleasurable distraction: if I'm thinking about someone else, I don't have to think about me. At the time of Leo's visits to Becky, my mum was battling cancer and I was well aware that apart from visiting, there was nothing I could do to help her, so I think I projected all that emotion onto my work with the children – where I could see good being achieved through the dogs' presence on the wards. I could do something for someone, if not myself. I could focus on Becky and, through Leo, see the positive transformation. I suppose what I'm saying is that I could offer hope in what looked like a hopeless situation.

It took me a long time to accept that all the dark thoughts and demons that I chose to internalise were still with me. I should have known that I could not hide them forever, but I couldn't have guessed that it would take a dog to heal me. That's why I can't help a tear pushing to the surface when I remember Becky and what she said about Leo as the dog who helped her to heal: '*I owe my life to Leo – and I always will.*'

For some, the intervention of a dog can be a bit of fun, for others it is a literal lifesaver. At the very least, dogs make everything better at the worst of times. And I should know.

4

Running dog lady!

IN 2008 SOUTHAMPTON CHILDREN'S HOSPITAL became my second home.

My youngest son, Ollie, was just nine years old when he was given a 65 per cent chance of recovery following his acute myeloid leukaemia diagnosis. I held on to that figure for dear life as our family and everything familiar to us at home was turned upside down. 'Don't google it, Lyndsey,' is what Mike said almost immediately after we had been given the diagnosis. He knew ... his medical training told him just how bad it could potentially be. Somehow, I didn't. Life moved so rapidly into our new routine.

Life certainly took a different shape after the diagnosis on 20 August 2008. Mike took compassionate leave for the first couple of months so that we could get our heads around what was happening. But, ever the surgeon, he wanted to continue supporting his colleagues, which meant spending some time in his office at the hospital working out what should happen with the patients he had booked for surgery. His dedication to his patients' welfare never shifted but, on this occasion, he simply couldn't put them first.

Mike and I took it day by day. We worked out which nights we would stay with Ollie and then our handover usually took place at lunchtime or mid-afternoon, depending on whether we were bringing our other son, 11-year-old Harry, in to visit his brother. Whoever was at home with Harry overnight took the dogs out first thing after taking Harry to the school bus and then sorted out stuff at home, including the myriad of cards, gifts and food parcels that were arriving from our truly kind friends and neighbours. The parent arriving at the hospital in the afternoon had a quick chat with the parent leaving, whose next job would be to either collect Harry from school en route to home or race to get to the bus stop so he could travel back home with his friends on the school bus.

The routine had to run like clockwork because that was the only way I could cope with my fear. I could lose Ollie. That fact never, for one second, left my head. Whatever I was doing, wherever I was, it was there. My auto-pilot-mum mode was switched on 24/7 and God help anyone who tried to turn down the speed or distract me from my routine.

Until that time, my only connection with Southampton Children's Hospital was that my husband worked there and I had also worked in the hospital's postgraduate medical centre for a short while before the boys were born. I considered our family very fortunate in many ways, one being that we were a fit and healthy lot. Just shows you how evil cancer is, waiting in the wings of life ready to invade the body of a nine-year-old boy.

Ollie's diagnosis came from nowhere: one minute we were all relaxing back at home after a fabulous family holiday in France and three days later, after feeling a bit unwell, Ollie was on the paediatric oncology ward receiving treatment and Mike and I were in discussions regarding his prognosis and short-term care. I was stunned, as if I had been hit on the head with a cricket bat. In fact, I wished that I had because nothing could have hurt me more than the words that came out of the paediatrician's mouth: 'I'm sorry to tell you that Oliver has leukaemia … the oncologist will come soon to discuss treatment with you …' I didn't hear the rest.

Mike deals with these people every day, he understands their language and hears the music behind their words. By the time the diagnosis came, it was late at night. I was aware of one thing: a medic talking to another medic will speak the un-sugared truth and so I knew that whatever Mike was being told it would be the whole truth and nothing but the truth and I was happy with that. I just didn't want to hear anymore.

Hospital shifts and anonymous patients had been the framework of our family life since I met Mike. Everything we arranged – children's appointments, family celebrations, holidays – was organised around surgical lists, meetings and medical conventions. I was the wife of a surgeon, all that went with the territory, but now we were just another set of parents with their very sick child, connected to all kinds of machinery in his hospital bed, and all I wanted to do was get on with making Ollie well again and get him home.

When I was the one at home, I loved to be out exercising our two dogs, Monty and Totty. Of course, those four-legged-friends never argued no matter how many miles I walked or ran with them to escape my fears over Ollie's prognosis. Little did anyone know that at that time it was the dogs, their peace and their companionship, that was holding me together.

I found out afterwards that some of the people from the village called me 'the running dog lady'. I earned the name because whenever I was seen in the village, I had Monty and then later our second dog, Totty, once she was old enough to join him at my heels. My motto prior to and during that time was: 'Gotta keep running or the demons will catch up!' I have a feeling that Monty in particular understood that need in me, because he never once complained or held back from a run, no matter what the weather dealt us; it had been the same since we began hitting the roads, paths and beaches to find some solace in this mad world. Monty had been my running partner for almost three years by the time of Ollie's diagnosis, sharing the miles; he probably knew me better than anyone.

I've always needed to keep busy and I love having a project on the go that I'm passionate about. My husband and sons would tell you that I'm better with something good to focus on and if it involves dogs, well, that's just perfect. Running became my 'keeping busy' and when Ollie was diagnosed I had already run the London Marathon the year before in aid of motor neurone disease. I had wanted to do it in memory of my grandfather who had suffered so horribly with the disease and the training just became what I did every morning with Monty, who was an enthusiastic running partner. Our vet was impressed with how we kept this big, solid, drooly food monster retriever on track with his weight – until I told him that we were in training for the Marathon and ten-mile runs were not unusual. It wasn't quite the same when we ran on the beach – thanks to the seagulls. Monty could never resist a seagull chase, so any other runners, or walkers, had to be on their guard to avoid being taken out by a whoosh of 'gold' as he zoomed back in to rejoin me on my run!

Apart from his usual sniff, think, pee moments en route, Monty was 'with' me all the way, keeping a bouncy pace matching me stride for stride, and I felt that he was keyed in to what was going on in my head too. He kept an eye on me. I swear that dog knew everything that there was to know about my feelings at the time – it was something special that we shared. We ran, I talked to him, we took moments when we stopped, just sitting on the pebbles staring out to sea ... He never argued or tried to move on or chase anything; he just went with the flow and if there were occasional tears, he was there to soak them up in his thick, golden coat.

Who would have thought that a golden retriever could be pet dog, running buddy, psychotherapist and best friend all rolled into one? But that was my first dog, Monty, and his closeness and understanding of me was never more valuable than when Ollie was in hospital.

Mike and I did alternate nights at the hospital so one of us was always with Ollie. It was the weirdest time of any day: with every fibre of your being, you wanted to be there in case anything happened and Ollie needed you, but there was always the feeling in the surreal hush that lingered in the corridors and the low hum of the monitors coming from each child's bay that nothing was going to happen to break the hypnotic state. The 'nothingness' was the most terrifying feeling of all.

I found it hard to sleep on some nights and that's when I felt an overwhelming desire to run. So, once I was sure Ollie was asleep, I left the ward and ran ... up and down the stairs from the children's oncology unit on the top floor down to the basement, and back again, over and over and over. It was more than just a need to get out of the ward for a few minutes to be alone: it was to escape an overwhelming feeling of helplessness. I couldn't fix this thing and I wanted to so very badly. My son was lying in a hospital bed, just yards from where I had been lying wide awake in the parents' bed, and I couldn't do a thing to take his cancer away. All I could do was trust in the experts and it was so hard. I wanted to shake my head and, like a kaleidoscope, shift the colours and mix the pieces around, change the picture in my mind. I didn't like the one that was there; I just couldn't make it go away. The nights I ran, I ran and ran, up and down, sometimes the sweat running down my face. I did it for myself so that I could be more present for Ollie.

I ran to stay sane.

I rarely met anyone while doing my stair-run very late at night or in the early hours of the morning, but I do remember meeting a security guard one night at the top of G-level staircase, just a short distance away from the doors of Piam Brown children's oncology ward. I reassured him that I was one of the parents of a child on the ward and he kindly suggested that I needed sleep too. It was around 4am and I knew that my night's sleep was already over, so I thanked him and headed back to check on Ollie before being first in the parents' shower room that morning.

Of course, it's perfectly reasonable for any of the night staff who popped up in the stairwell to be passed by this sweaty runner wearing either a frown or tears to think I was mad. Maybe I was a little bit mad: I certainly would have been if I'd sat on the ward in the same place, wide awake, waiting for something or nothing to happen. It's the worst situation in the world for a 'fixer' to be stuck in a place where they can't 'fix'.

While Ollie slept, the running kept me fit and it gave me the space to think. And it was in the silent, semi-gloom of the hospital staircase, in the early hours of one morning in early September 2008, that I made a deal with myself: that if Ollie recovered fully then I would give back. I just hadn't worked out exactly how I would do it.

5

Animal Assisted Intervention?

ONE TIME IN THE MIDDLE OF THE NIGHT, in his room, I stood with my thoughts for a few moments, illuminated by the pulse of blue light, this time from an ambulance pulling into one of the bays at the back of the hospital immediately below. Everything was lost in the blue, as I imagined the scene of my own worst-case scenario: the hustle of paramedics surrounding a young patient, the hunched parent or carer, one hand grasping the trolley as it is wheeled at speed into the neurological emergency department. I thought of the patient's pain and the relatives' fear in that moment and felt grateful. I knew what we faced with Ollie: where the problem lay, what could be done, what would happen if he made it and if he did not. Mike and I had discussed how lucky we were that he did not need 'repairing' like a patient would do if they were involved in a major accident. Parents of children with major trauma have no idea what is ahead for them, no idea how their lives will have already changed beyond all recognition, or how they will grieve for the life they were promised with their child, a life that has now gone.

Now, when I think back to that night and my fear in that blur of blue, I can't help remembering a young patient called Felix, who I met with Leo seven years later ...

It was in October 2015 that the Hampshire and Isle of Wight Air Ambulance delivered Felix to waiting Emergency Department staff at Southampton Hospital – it was less than an hour after he forgot to take his sport shoes to school. No doubt he shouted 'bye' to his mum as he grabbed his bag and headed out of the house, eager to be where he needed to be on time, looking forward to a day ahead which always included sport at his high level of competition. He would have had a million things on his mind, including a quick rundown of what he had stuffed into his sports bag. Shoes? No, of all the things to leave behind! Felix turned for home.

He wouldn't have seen the car. It hit him right outside his house. He had serious head injuries, his legs were smashed and later it was found even his vocal chords were damaged. The full consequences of the accident were, at first, unknown, but life changed in seconds for 11-year-old Felix, an aspiring Team GB triathlete. That day changed his life, his dreams, and it changed everything for his parents and sisters too. Felix was rushed into hospital and ultimately into paediatric intensive care, where he was put into an induced coma. A few days later I first met him and his traumatised parents at his bedside.

Leo and I visited Felix many times as he moved from intensive care to the high-dependency unit and ultimately to his single room on the general ward just up the corridor from some of our other patients. In the early days we just visited during Felix's brief periods of wakefulness so he could feel Leo's soft fur between his fingers, to give him something different and comforting to focus on while his head injury started to heal. They were also moments when I could offer whichever parent was with him a chance to chat about something other than hospitals before saying our goodbyes until the next time.

With every visit I saw Felix making slow but steady progress through his early rehab. Considering the huge physical trauma that he'd endured it was no surprise that belief in his resilience and bravery were well established with the staff. His broken bones were mendable, Mike and his many surgical colleagues took care of that, and eventually, he was out of plaster but still very wobbly on his legs, with lots of healing still to do.

One particular day when we visited Felix I'm convinced Leo realised that he needed to put on a bit of a show if he was going to really help this brave young man. Like a boxer entering the ring for a heavyweight title fight, Leo strutted his stuff into the room just when Felix had decided he wasn't keen on yet another physio session. Thankfully, we arrived at the right time as a session involving Leo had been planned by Kate, his physiotherapist. We escorted him in his wheelchair, pushed by his dad, down to the main physiotherapy department where Felix, directed and supported by Kate and her assistant, Liv, was encouraged to stand, reach up to the sky and lean down towards Leo, who was lying on the floor. Core strength was the aim that day and while Felix was unsteady at first, his determination never wavered ... He wanted to give Leo either a stroke on the head when he reached down or the treat that I passed him every second stretch.

The hand-eye and physical coordination required to take the treat from my hand into his, hold it while he stretched both arms up to the sky, then leaned forward and stretched down to feed it to Leo lying waiting for it was extraordinary. It would require much concentration from anyone, let alone someone who had recently suffered brain and physical injuries. Determined as always, Felix, with the mind of an athlete, was there in front of us. The more he did, the more he wanted to do, as Leo lay there waiting for him. I looked around the room and everyone was smiling. Another physio team had appeared at the door and Felix's dad captured a video to share with their family and friends. I smiled at Leo, my four-legged physio assistant. I realised later that what we had done in that session was create some true Animal Assisted Therapy (AAT). I showed the video to Mike when he came home and he was astonished, not just at how well Felix had done but at how Leo lay so patiently, as though he understood the job in hand. Of course, he did ... Leo's intuition was on full-power that day.

On another visit, Felix's look of smiley surprise said it all as Leo made his presence felt and gave a giant tail wag to say: 'Hello, I'm back!' Having been in so many times, Leo knew exactly where to find Felix on the ward – just along the corridor from Dylan, Archie and Sophie, to name but a few of our long-termers who were there at that time.

The dogs always cause a bit of a stir when they arrive on the children's wards because almost everyone is pleased to see them and you can feel their presence triggering a ripple of excitement and anticipation along the corridors. It's a really powerful response and one that Leo soaks up with a giddy appreciation. I sometimes feel like I'm a minder for a Hollywood film star! Leo greets every patient with a swagger and a smile; it's just his laid-back, cheeky way, but I really do think he can sense when a little extra charm is needed to help build the bridge between a patient. This came through in Felix's care.

Like all patients with multiple rehab requirements, Felix had a weekly diary pinned to the wall detailing when to expect visits from his physio, occupational therapist and speech therapist, amongst others, and the intermittent trips back to theatre for operations to advance his recovery from some of his multiple injuries. It was one of the busiest timetables I've ever seen, so, unless we had been asked to assist in any of the sessions, it was a bit of a challenge to time our visits so that we didn't interrupt anything.

On one day we were just arriving as the speech therapist was leaving. Felix looked up and smiled, pleased to see us, and held his hand out towards Leo, who was quick to move in for the fuss. While Leo did his meet and greet stuff, I asked the speech therapist if there was anything we could do to help Felix while we were there. I've got to admit that I was over the moon when she said that perhaps we could help him by practising his exhaling (puffing) exercises. Once I'd clarified with her what we were trying to achieve, Felix demonstrated 'puffing'; it was barely audible. Then it hit me: 'Well, that sounds like Leo when he pants, Felix! I'm sure we can help you with that.'

The therapist left and Felix was ready for a little break so we chatted a bit, with Felix mouthing some words that I did my best to understand. Over our time together I learnt to listen to his very faint words as well as trying to lipread. Like his parents and the staff caring for him, most of us who had known Felix for a while could make out what he was trying to say and with me it was usually something cheeky about the dog, so he'd be all smiles when I got it right!

Stroking Leo for about ten minutes as we chatted gave Felix time to rest his vocal chords and during that time I had an idea. When I said that I was going to get Leo to do the 'puffing' exercise, naturally he looked a bit confused. I looked out of the door to his room and saw an empty corridor. 'Wait there ...' I said. 'I'll be back in a minute!' I left the room with Leo in tow and told the nurse at the nurses' station opposite that, while the corridor was empty, I was about to run up and down it and then she'd understand why. Not wanting to waste the opportunity, I took off at a sprint, along with a very bewildered-looking Leo, past the nine rooms along the short stretch of corridor and back again, with parents looking on from their children's rooms. The nurse in charge smiled and I heard her say to one of the watching parents: 'Oh, don't worry, you might think she looks like a madwoman but I think I know what she's up to.' I could hear the tittering at my expense, but I got what I wanted.

I sat Leo in front of Felix and said: 'Look, he's doing what you need to do! Do you think you can do it at the same time as Leo?' Poor Felix gave blowing-out all the puff he could muster but Leo's noisy panting was drowning out his faint breaths! 'OK, a rethink is needed here. Felix, how about Leo does his puff then you do yours? That would work and you would have to get in between each of Leo's breath sounds. Shall we give it a try? Leo's ready ...'

Felix repeated it a few times with Leo playing his part and no idea of what he was achieving with his very loud panting! We were having great fun with something that we could carry on practising over the next few visits with the full blessing of the speech therapist. The panting metronome ... who knew a dog could help with speech therapy?

Nothing moves too quickly with rehab; it is mostly a mix of try, repeat, review, do, repeat, review, all combined with a huge dose of patience. Leo and I were invited to work with Felix sometimes because it was clear our patient connected Leo with having fun. Funny how the presence of a smiley dog can be such a useful workmate. As Felix slowly recovered, it seemed so unfair to me that here was a boy who was doing so well despite so many injuries but, just as his concentration was improving alongside his limb movement, his voice couldn't really be heard. It must have been so hard for his family at times as they longed for their gifted triathlete to recover from this awful accident.

I had another idea; I woke up in the night thinking about it. It's strange thinking back to that time now because the words Animal Assisted Intervention (AAI) meant nothing to me then. There was no eureka moment where I found myself saying: 'Oh, I'm using AAI here!' It dawned on me gradually that what I was doing on my visits had a proper name. Reading more and more about the power of the human-animal bond and its therapeutic benefits, I discovered how dogs (and other animals, such as horses) can 'intervene' in a patient's rehabilitation in such a positive way. That gradual personal discovery was part of our journey with Felix. When we gained the support of his speech therapist it made me want to try something new on our next visit.

That morning, when I came down to let the dogs out – at this point I had four, including Jessie, who you will hear more of later – I checked that they could all sit to a hand signal. Leo did it immediately – the others just ignored me, wondered what on earth could be more important than the first sniff of morning air outside, and bounced out of the dog flap I had just opened! Poor Leo sat there looking confused as he looked at the tails of the other three heading out. He was not entirely impressed with the impromptu 6.30am training session. But I couldn't stop there. Out on our walk at the country park I stopped them all every now and then along the way using just a hand signal, not a voice command and, one by one, they all remembered what I wanted them to do – to 'sit'! 'Very impressive,' said one of the regular walkers we used to pass most mornings as she walked by with Freddie, her elderly Dalmatian.

Monty, Totty, Jessie and Leo sat there looking at me and I willed them not to move. It was lucky it was only Freddie passing us. Had it been one of the younger dogs that played with them, it would have been a different matter and not impressive at all. Still, I only needed one of them to do it at the hospital and when they have their working jacket on, they are usually reliable.

We carried on like that over the next few days until it was time to visit Felix again. The dogs probably thought I was getting a bit obsessive, and maybe I was, but they were due a refresher course anyway. No one on the wards wants to hear a woman nagging her dog, especially if we are being asked to wait while the patient is having instructions from one of the healthcare professionals. We always have to be on our best behaviour because we are guests on the wards. This was good timing to get them all up to speed on a basic command. I didn't need to worry about Leo. He was, as always, paying attention.

Our next visit provided the moment of truth. Could I combine hand signals with Felix's vocal exercises? Only one way to find out. Felix was up for a chat with the dog and Leo thought anything involving Felix was great fun, so it was game on!

Felix and Leo greeted each other with their usual mutual smiles and I could tell that Felix was curious to try out the new idea as I explained it to him, so after a little bit of chat, I suggested that he tried to tell Leo to sit. He mouthed, at the lowest possible volume, 'sit' but all I heard was the 't' and so I gave a discreet hand signal to Leo. As the dog sat, Felix absolutely beamed with pride. 'Well done,' I said. 'That was brilliant! Leo can hear you because he has super-special canine hearing but it is still a bit hard for me to hear, so can we try again?' This time I positioned myself so Leo could see both me and Felix and again the dog sat as instructed – with some more discreet hand signalling from me, of course. We repeated this a few more times and it was so much fun and so wonderful to see Felix's pride in his results. It must have been lovely for him to issue instructions after so many months of receiving them.

That day I walked out of the hospital feeling ten feet tall. My idea had worked! I had again created something bespoke for a specific patient and I gave Leo the biggest hug when we got back to the car because I really could not have done it without him. Driving home, I could feel my smile spreading from ear to ear and I was once again bursting to tell Mike that evening all about our new breakthrough with Felix. Fortunately, because Mike was one of his surgeons, this was a patient we could discuss without breaching confidentiality, so as soon as he came through the front door, I started gabbling on about Leo and how Felix had reacted. That was such a big moment for me.

Mike had initially been a bit sceptical about how the dogs could help his patients, but only because, as he used to say: 'I know what our dogs get up to and how mucky they can get!' I knew what he meant, but all of those fears had been allayed by what had been agreed with the infection control team at the hospital and I always ensured that the dog was washed, dried and brushed before heading into the hospital environment. Thankfully Mike's scepticism didn't hold us back as Professor Clarke, his senior colleague in the department, had encountered therapy dogs working with children in the USA when he'd been lecturing there and was happy for us to be on his ward. When Mike heard about the speech therapy with hand signals, even he had to admit this was another triumph for Leo, for Felix of course, and for me. It has always meant everything to have my husband's support and his blessing.

That first chance meeting with the speech therapist as she was leaving Felix's room was the first time another allied health professional had acknowledged that we might help their patient. We had already worked with some of the inpatients alongside their doctors, nurses, physiotherapists and occupational therapists, but this felt like things were expanding into different spheres. I'm not sure that I had read anything in my books about therapy dogs supporting patients through speech therapy at that stage; I think that came almost instinctively from me. You see, I felt with a clear, deep conviction that I could help, and that help had to be something simple and dog-friendly.

Felix saw a therapy dog during his stay about three times a week, sometimes just to drop in to say hello with a smile and check how he was getting on, and other times as part of his therapy. Mostly Leo, but the other members of the team also visited, and this helped Felix with memory and recognition and, over time, he was able to name each of the dogs who had visited him.

As his confidence grew and his speech developed, Felix began to tell Leo to 'down' (lie down), 'sit', 'stand'. Later, when he was practising his hand coordination, he passed a ball to Leo at first and then graduated to throwing it, asking him to retrieve it and then 'drop' (the ball).

Eventually, after months and months, it was time for Felix to start walking outside again and of course this meant passing cars as they drove around the hospital roads. Felix had walked a good distance inside the hospital but his physiotherapist wanted us to go on his first longer walk, including a stroll outside. It was a cold day, and to be honest, I didn't think we would get far. Felix was wrapped up warmly in his outdoor clothes and fleece as he walked, pausing from time to time to lean against Kate, his physio. Felix's dad pushed a wheelchair ahead of them in case it was needed and I walked beside Felix and Kate as they took each step forward with him, looking into the distance and then occasionally looking down at Leo. Felix was holding Leo's patient lead, I had the other one in my hand and we chatted about dog things as we walked.

After a while, I felt frozen, wearing just a polo shirt and skirt, but nothing was going to make me stop this amazing session even if I was shivering. I almost expected a round of applause from the gaggle of smokers in their surgical gowns and dressing gowns as we passed them very slowly. 'What a lovely dog,' one of them said as we passed. I wondered if that helped Felix as he knew they were looking at the dog and not at him, but of course it didn't matter. The important thing was, Felix was back on his feet. It took so much concentration for those previously injured legs to walk every step but walk they did, and with Leo as his companion, he walked from the door at one end of the hospital to the entrance at the other. It was a huge distance for Felix and more than had been expected of him. Pride radiated from Felix's dad, Kate his physiotherapist, and of course, me. Felix looked so pleased with himself.

Once home (and thawed out), I was buzzing with excitement! I knew that Leo's patience and eagerness to please was a big part of something healing, something incredible, and I was so proud of him. He showed that the presence of a therapy dog in rehabilitation can make such a positive difference and the rush of pride, when it goes so well, can lift any gloomy, cold day.

Leo, the fun companion, the distraction, the bridge to healing, made it fun for all of us. And it worked for Felix because he loved dogs and he especially enjoyed being with Leo.

6

Hospital mum mode

I WAS STILL AT THE WINDOW when the ambulance pulled slowly and silently away, taking with it the stress-inducing pulse of blue light. I had scared myself enough for one night, just imagining how much worse things could be for us. I turned to look at Ollie lying in his bed sleeping while the drugs surged through the tubes entering his body and hoped they were doing their work.

I returned to my bed, which had been placed beside Ollie's, to try to get some sleep. He was still sleeping peacefully. I wanted to put my hand on my son's head but I didn't want to risk waking him. There were many moments like that over days and nights spent at his bedside. During the day patients snatched only occasional bits of sleep between treatment, visits and observations, making a night's sleep so valuable. There were times when I felt truly alone, the nights being the worst of all. I could get to sleep but found it hard to stay asleep most nights. Wanting to be there for Ollie was paramount, but I also wanted to be anywhere that was silent and where I could truly relax, something that is actually impossible if you are the parent of a child in hospital. His pumps and machines made relatively quiet noises that he seemed able to sleep through but they jarred me back to wakefulness and, if I did make it to a deep sleep, they woke me like a cruel reminder of where we were ... and why.

The role of the parent on duty at the hospital was simply to roll with the punches. Whatever was happening to Ollie that day was all that mattered, that and the struggle to avoid looking too concerned or confused when new information came your way. Now I always tell people to ask questions but not to worry if they can't remember the answers because the staff will always tell you what you need to know when you need to know it. For the first month or so that Ollie was on the oncology ward, I remember being amazed at how many parents could name the drugs their child was on and some would ask which drugs he was being treated with as if they wanted to compare. I felt very awkward in the early days when I couldn't even remember what day it was, let alone the name of the medication being pumped into him. But it didn't take long, certainly by the time Ollie was on his second month of chemo, I could name his drugs and when they were due too. When I visit oncology patients now, I always joke with parents at the beginning of their journey that they mustn't worry if they can't remember everything they've been told because by the time their child's treatment is over they will have memorised every single detail – and will never forget them.

No one wants to find themselves the parent with a child in a hospital environment, that's the one thing we all have in common, that and the knowledge that we're all in this together, making the best of a terrifying situation. We don't want to wander too far from our child's bedside – and I always wanted to be ready to entertain Ollie if he was up to it – but beyond the confines of our individual rooms we were respectfully aware of the desperation of other parents. We generally collide with each other in the coffee room or parents' bathroom, and there's always plenty of interaction with the ward staff as they regularly come in and out to check, inform and reassure. Conversation is optional, that's an unwritten rule, but there's also a universal acceptance that we are all invisibly reaching out to each other with an offer to listen, to talk, do whatever we can to support each other in our shared, other-worldly experience. Sometimes the offer of a listening ear is all that's needed and that can happen as you pass each other in the parents' lounge or make another caffeine infusion in the ward kitchen. Suddenly, people you would never have met in ordinary life become your confidantes, sharing a similar burden that very few parents will, thankfully, ever understand: the burden of looking like it's all completely doable.

Home and my gorgeous dogs became a super-sanctuary for me. Loneliness in hospital was one thing but home was isolating, too. It wasn't anyone's fault; it was just a case of once the daily practical stuff was ticked off my list, my mind couldn't switch off. I was living two lives: one at home and another at the hospital, and the thoughts of both were whirring around in my head wherever I was. I think the dogs keyed into my need big-time and made a determined pact to fill that lonely void by sticking to me like blobs of glue.

When Harry and I reached home in the evenings Monty and Totty greeted us with their usual 'Yay, you're back! We love you so much, you guys!' They launched themselves towards us like we had returned from years away, not just a few hours since being left for the early-afternoon change of parent at the hospital. We welcomed their unconditional love with open arms. As the dogs settled, Harry usually went off to get his homework out of the way before supper and I stayed to play with the dogs for half an hour or so in the garden. They loved that fun time with their toys but probably because they knew it was food time next.

As I cooked our supper, I'd listen to the many messages on the answerphone, all enquiring about Ollie, some asking how we were all coping, all sending their best wishes. I've never really got over how wonderful people were to us at that difficult time. There was so much kindness around us and I wanted to get back to everyone right away but I admit that fatigue got the better of me most evenings.

We were a couple of weeks into our visiting routine when two of our very good friends started to take on the role of our 'school gate informers', which was a great relief. Social media was in its infancy then, so their help updating well-wishers was great because it was impossible to speak to everyone personally, or for the parent on the hospital shift to make calls with Ollie in earshot. There was no way I wanted to let him hear exactly how worried I was.

I loved the early-evening relaxation at home with Harry and the dogs. I had never appreciated our home so much as

I did over that time. Just to be back in my own environment with the door shut and no one around us hovering to take a temperature, check a line or do any number of other bits and pieces the wonderful hospital staff had to all the time in order to care for our son. Much as I loved being on the ward for Ollie, I also needed some time with Harry and the dogs – a little time, just to be normal. And to go to the loo without having to rush in case I'd missed something or a member of the clinical team needed to explain something. Funny how, in extraordinary times, you come to value the mundane things in life.

Supper with Harry was always special and he had taken to chatting about his day at his new school while I opened the post, which quickly began to include a rush of 'get well soon' cards interspersed with the usual bills of life. Once we had finished eating, Harry was usually keen to escape to a computer game, so I launched into returning some of the messages on the answerphone and that's how the evenings went, alongside the usual stuff like sorting washing, compiling things that needed to go back to the hospital the following day: clothes, books, toys, some of the cards and gifts that had been sent to our home. Once Harry was in bed and the chores all done the evenings seemed to disappear.

All I wanted to do then was chat with Mike ... but I couldn't. As weird as this may sound, we agreed that the one at home would wait for the parent at the hospital to call home once Ollie had gone to sleep. It seemed the right thing to do because time with Ollie in the evening was often spent watching a film, playing and chatting, so a call was likely to intrude on all of that. So, unless Ollie had a burning desire to bid me goodnight, there was no call until he was asleep.

The time between Harry going to bed and Mike's call could sometimes be a couple of hours, which I'd spend wide awake, running over potential topics of conversation in my head, and feeling desperate to chat. Mike and I were passing like ships in the night, rarely together in the same place, which made this end-of-day conversation so special, so important to both of us. Thinking back, it must have been a pretty unsettling time for the dogs who, I now realise, must have picked up on the strong vibes of restlessness that I was giving off as I tried to think of things to distract myself while I waited. It was too late in the evening to call friends or family so, as my batteries began to run down, I realised that the best thing to do was give in to the two golden retrievers who were beside me, following me around trying to persuade me to ... sit down with them.

So, there we were, side by side on the lounge floor with my back against the sofa – me in the middle – the TV providing some unidentifiable background babble to fill the empty silence in the house and the anxious whirring in my head. Monty and Totty snuggled into me, him resting his head on my lap and Totty lying on her back, as close as she could, just willing me to stroke her belly. Both positioned as if to say: 'Come on, Mum ... keep stroking, you know how this works ...' There's no way to resist my dogs when they want to give or receive attention because they just don't give up on you; one way or another, they draw you into their version of relaxation, which usually involves lying down and snoring. On those evenings, they probably wondered why I was being so needy.

I had no reason to argue with what Monty and Totty decided was good for me. Sitting with them, stroking and talking to them, telling them my secret thoughts and trusting in their silence gave me moments of complete peace. The only noise that could break the stillness was the phone, which always startled me but I'd rush to grab it, even though I sometimes feared what the voice on the other end would say.

Chatting with Mike was always a massive relief. Sometimes, not always, my emotions would get the better of me and when they did the dogs immediately sat up and offered their paws. Monty was adept at giving both paws, thanks to the many hours of 'training' with treats that had been put in by the boys! I think he loved the round of applause they gave him every time Monty did 'the double'! I happily took their outstretched paws as an offer of a hug, which I readily accepted, and those wonderful dogs never withdrew from me. Monty had a sweet way of offering and swapping paws, so if my voice trembled or I became anxious, he lifted his left paw, then the right and then both … all I could do was smile. There he was, just five years old, and Totty just over 12 months, giving me all the moves they had to make me happy. Mike and I always ended our conversations on a high to put the positive back into our world, then bade each other goodnight before I put the dogs to bed.

It was usually around midnight before I made it upstairs. Sleep came very quickly. Although I was uncomfortably alone in our lovely bed, its softness was a welcome retreat from the world. The house was silent and I could afford to slip into a deep sleep, knowing that I was home and I didn't have to catnap for Ollie's sake, but something always managed to wake me at the annoying time of three or four in the morning: far too early to get up or even let the dogs out. I lay there, unable to phone Mike as I wanted him to sleep and certainly didn't want to disturb Ollie. But once awake, trying to get back to sleep was pointless and I realised that the hours ahead involved just me, alone with my thoughts. I didn't want to burden anyone else; that wouldn't have been fair and besides I was more fortunate than most as I had two faithful dogs downstairs.

The first time I pulled on my dressing gown in the early hours and headed down the stairs in the dark, I wondered if Monty and Totty would be awake. Silly me, of course they were and their eyes shone out of the gloom to meet mine. I could tell from their puzzled expressions that they were curious about what I was up to and why was I wandering about in the middle of the night. I opened the kitchen door so they could come through to join me as I sat on the bottom stair in the dark hallway. They both leant into me and snuggled up, ready to listen to all I had to share with them. They knew. They knew me. I stroked them and chatted just as though I was talking to a counsellor. But they were better than any professional 'listener'; they had all the natural empathy of a wise and trusted friend wrapped in that most valuable of gifts – unconditional love.

I told them everything that I was worried about – Ollie's prognosis, my feelings of inadequacy in the face of leukaemia and of not being enough for my sons and my husband. I kept talking as my golden companions listened to my brain dump, soaking up every word as I stroked them. They soon returned to sleep but that didn't matter to me, they were still physically present. Sitting with them, I sometimes entered an almost hypnotic state of peace and calm.

Soon it would be 6am and time to open the dog flap, to start another day. Very soon I'd hear Harry getting ready to come down for breakfast and then, just over an hour later, I would take him to catch the school bus. Then it was time for the dogs to have their run and that's when I felt the tiredness leave my body to be replaced by a rush of adrenaline in preparation for that day's battles, whatever they turned out to be. After a shower, followed by checking in on my small business and the colleagues running it while I couldn't be there, food shopping and general faffing around, I was out of the house by early afternoon and into our hospital visiting cycle. This time it would be Mike heading back home ... And so it went on.

Without doubt, Monty and Totty deserved their early breakfast, after their night as canine counsellors.

Our time while Ollie was in hospital was full on and I'd say that it was busiest, in many ways, for the parent on the home run. Our focus was, inevitably, on Ollie, but Harry was only 11 years old and he needed us, too. He had just started at senior school and was loving it, but of course having a sibling admitted to hospital two weeks before term started didn't make the move to a new environment any easier. Added to that, we knew that Harry was missing his younger brother, so the visiting routine had to have all that built in – or so we assumed. It turned out that we had overthought it all and although he wanted to see Ollie, Harry didn't always know what to say and he also had homework to do. So, a couple of weeks into this intense routine we realised that we needed to focus on both of our sons as individuals. In short, Harry needed to get home after school and do his homework rather than go into the hospital every evening.

This realisation shook a few old niggles to the surface, like the time Harry eventually admitted that most of the Sunday mornings he had spent on a muddy rugby pitch were mornings he would rather have spent elsewhere. That conversation came not long after he won a silver medal at the Concept2 indoor rowing championships, after which he was offered the opportunity to try out river rowing at Canford school near Wimborne. The coach, Ian Dryden, offered to teach Harry as part of his community club that was attached to the boarding school. So, in September, two weeks after Ollie had been diagnosed, I called Ian to explain what was happening and said that while the evenings were still light, Harry would love to come down after school and have a go. He started the following Monday.

I arranged for my parents to do Monday afternoons with Ollie so that I could leave the hospital in time to go home, get my running kit on, grab Monty and Totty and some food for Harry, before racing back to the school to collect him. If we managed a quick getaway, we could be in Wimborne by 5pm and Harry would be straight on the water. It was our time together to chat about his day at his new senior school, just the two of us – and the dogs in the back of the car. I was excited for Harry, who was now doing the thing he loved and once he was in his boat and on the river, I collected the dogs from the car and set off running along the riverbank with them. It was bliss; fresh air, no hospital smells or sounds. I felt at ease again and like I didn't have to be on the alert for this tiny speck of time.

There was an ease in knowing that as Harry took the oars to begin rowing up and down the river, Mike would be back at Ollie's bedside and I could allow myself to enjoy this time without feeling guilty. What I had not anticipated was how animated Harry would be after the rowing. It was as if he came alive out on the water! He absolutely loved it. I remember telling Mike on the evening after the first rowing trip how I thought Harry had found his passion and indeed it turned out to be the sport that dominated his teenage years. I loved the fact we were doing it just for him – no poorly sibling, no hospital ties, just me and him doing something he wanted to do – and we had managed to manipulate the routine to make it possible.

The rowing trips were good for us and the dogs were loving it too; all that water and running not to mention the 'tea break' at the end! Ian was brilliant with Harry, so relaxed and kind and always ready to offer us tea or coffee in the boathouse on a help-yourself basis, which was just brilliant. A mish-mash of cups, coffee, milk, etc., all there on the workbench next to a rigger jigger and a few oily rags. A blessed far cry from the cleanliness of the hospital kitchen where everyone had their own things in the fridge, plastered in name stickers to make sure we all took responsibility for the food we took in to tempt our sick child to eat. Always, when we left the boathouse at the end of a session, Harry's hunger would flare up big time, so a visit to McDonald's drive-thru at Ferndown became part of our trip. It was a treat we both looked forward to and enjoyed together on the 39-mile journey home.

The dogs loved those Monday evenings on the river, especially Totty, who didn't need any encouragement to jump into the water. Despite my efforts to keep her out, if she fancied it, she always managed to find a way through the reeds and launched herself in with a great splosh! Both of them were usually very well-behaved and just ran along the towpath with me, passing the cows grazing in the fields nearby, smiling at the walkers we passed and loving the fresh air, but sometimes the water was too much of a call on their canine senses. I just had to make sure that they stayed away from the boats and that Totty didn't try to join Harry onboard!

Sadly, week by week, the time got shorter as the evenings closed in, forcing the move to Saturday mornings. It didn't really matter, when we got used to it, as it was still a relief not to be tethered to the hospital just for that brief weekly episode. The feeling of freedom and that time with Harry has stayed with me. We needed that, all of us, and so did Monty and Totty. The entire hospital experience gave us not only a different routine – it became a 'lifestyle' packed with emotional stress that was split dramatically between the alien austerity of the hospital and the welcome comfort of home.

Time spent with Ollie made us believe that nothing bad could happen to him while we were there. In some supernatural, helicopter parent fashion we wouldn't allow it as long as one of us was hovering close. For me, our routine was working like clockwork and its rhythmic certainty kept me feeling that I was in a safe place. A few days at home every month between each cycle of chemo and then we started again. As long as I knew what was going on then everything was OK and the rejigging of the plans to get things right for Harry felt like a massive relief.

The rowing sessions were working fine for everyone and that included Totty. While Ollie was in hospital, Harry, being the only child consistently at home, was the most constant companion for Totty. She was just 14 months old when Ollie was admitted and I was glad she had Monty at home with her for the few hours when there was no human company there. At least Monty knew his family were usually more reliable and available. She was still learning lots and getting through the leggy puppy stage – a bit like 11-year-old Harry! She loved being outdoors and those rowing trips were heaven to her. She adored Harry and seemed to hone in on his need for a friend to lean on while his brother was away. Happy to fill that gap, Totty must have seen Harry as the most reliable human being in her life because he was the one who always came home to her. One or other of the adults came home but Harry was always there, no matter what. In turn, I guess Totty was Harry's constant at a very unsettling time for him.

Later, in his teens, when Harry rowed with the Leander team at Henley, he was away for weekends and I would occasionally notice Totty sniff the car door handle on the passenger side when I returned after dropping him off. I often wondered whether she did this to remind her of his scent for the short time he was away.

Occasionally I took the dogs with me to collect Harry from Henley on Sunday mornings and we often ran along the riverbank there while waiting for his training session to end. I'm sure what Totty really wanted was to join him on the water, as she'd often attempted to do in the early days and I still find that need to be close to Harry a very touching feature of their special bond, which lasted her lifetime. Be it nature or nurture, Totty, the whirlwind puppy, with the fabulous swishy tail, was always the independent one and in many ways that complemented Monty's sleepy, 'needy' personality. After all, Monty and I were bonded from day one and he had become my rock in all of this terrifying hospital stuff.

7

'I'd rather die ...'

OLLIE HAD BEEN IN HOSPITAL about three weeks when he tore away the line feeding the drugs into his body. Frustrated with how he was feeling and the confines of his hospital bed while his friends were at home enjoying their week-ends, our son blurted out: 'I'd rather die than not see the dogs again.' I was out running with Monty and Totty when Mike rang to tell me. The words were a dagger to my heart. There we were, thinking that we had everything balanced and there was Ollie, the young lad at the centre of this awful time, missing the one thing that the rest of us were so lucky to have on tap – the comforting companionship of the dogs.

What could I do?

I carried on running towards home. We were nearly there. Dogs were a strict 'no-no' on paediatric oncology back in 2008 and when my husband called me to say what had happened, I didn't even contemplate asking if I could break that rule. Up to then, I had never even encountered therapy dogs. All I knew was that I wanted Ollie to see our dogs. And surely there had to be a way to get around this. After all, who would it offend? And think of the joy that a pair of golden visitors would bring. My 'fixer' mode was immediately switched into overdrive.

By the time we arrived back home, I had formulated an idea. I knew Southampton Children's Hospital pretty well by then so how close could I get the dogs to Ollie without breaking the rules? Or maybe I needed to look at this from another angle – how close could Mike get Ollie, in a wheelchair, to the dogs?

We already knew that the drugs line couldn't be reinserted until later in the day, so it was a great opportunity to give Ollie some time away from the ward. In my head, I did a quick mental recce of the building – its exits and entrances, windows and car parks – and then it hit me. I could take the dogs in the car and walk them to the staff car park at the back of the hospital, which would be less busy as it was a Sunday afternoon. I put the dogs in the car and rang Mike to say I was coming. He told me he had the nursing sister's permission to take Ollie off the ward but only for a short period of time. Mike suggested we keep it a surprise in case I was delayed for any reason en route. I leapt in the car, still sweaty from my run but eager to get there as soon as we could.

I parked up and hurriedly got the dogs out of the back of the car. They were keen to have a good old sniff around the new territory, that is until they walked around the corner and sniffed ... Ollie! Noses in the air, they accelerated when they saw him. I shrieked with excitement. Relieved, excited and with a few tears, I watched Ollie's super-surprised expression when he saw the dogs. He was beaming with delight and thanks to his hands being in protective surgical gloves, he was able to hold the dogs' leads as they pulled him around in his chariot with me taking a grainy video on my phone. A video that I now hold very dear: it reminds me of yet another special time when Monty and Totty made a huge difference to our lives. It was a little bit of normality, a family enjoying time with their dogs – it just happened to be in a hospital car park! With the gloves on his hands, he was also able to stroke the dogs. It wasn't normal, but then nor was anything else at that time. It was close enough for the reconnection to be made with Ollie and in his smiles we saw a reminder that our dogs were there for all of us, inside and outside the hospital. We just needed to find a way of making sure, for as long as this new episode was to last, that no one was ever left out.

I remember standing at the window listening to Ollie's breathing as he slept in his room with the chemo surging down the tubes and through him. I hoped that he was slowly having his cancerous cells eradicated, but only his final bone marrow biopsy right at the end of his treatment would tell us whether they had completely disappeared. Until that time there were many, many more courses of chemo and the occasional setback, including a nerve-racking period when Ollie was unable to see for a few days and his eyes gave him terrible pain, which required morphine to keep it under control until it was resolved. Nothing in healthcare is entirely straightforward and we certainly learnt that during his treatment.

We were lucky we knew the nature of our fight; we could focus on that. Obviously, acute myeloid leukaemia was not what we would have chosen for anyone, let alone one of our sons, but it wasn't the worst diagnosis because we saw a way ahead. The really scary thing about it all was how life with cancer became our new 'normal'. I didn't like it but I found a way to work with it – but of course that was only because I couldn't change it.

Hopes to have Ollie home for Christmas were dashed when he suffered a setback, which meant it was January before we were finally allowed to take him home to recuperate. He still had his central line in with a clamp attached so that his treatment could quickly restart, should anything change. That would only be removed at the end of February if all went well over the following few weeks. The responsibility of ensuring the line didn't get damaged was a huge one for me now that he was home. I had been shown how the clamp must remain attached at all times and I was given the number to call if I had any concerns. We were home and life was different.

The optimist in me felt that we were finally released from cancer's hold on our family and at last we were able to return to our life on 'normal' street. In my mind we had endured almost five months of living in a parallel universe, forced to outwit an invisible enemy that had taken hold of Ollie and who at times we feared would refuse to give him back. I decided that from then on things were going to be all about our family, and that included the amazing Monty and Totty.

Of course, in reality, we weren't free of leukaemia's hold on us, not yet, but Ollie was home. As his strength began to return, he was keener than ever to get outside with the dogs, although sometimes he thought he had more energy than he could actually muster. His energy recovery came slowly, in fits and bursts, and although we couldn't risk anything too strenuous, whenever he was up to it, we headed for the prom at Lee-on-Solent beach, where he walked a little with Monty and Totty. Once the dogs had done an energetic seagull chase as well as all their sniffing and 'stuff', Monty offered himself up as Ollie's leaning post, hairy support and comfort blanket. Watching the dogs and the boys together, there was no doubt in my mind that Monty and Totty missed having their little buddies around and were keen to be around them. When Ollie first came home they swished their tails around him, nuzzled him in their welcome back to the safety of the pack. Their curious snouts sniffed a bit when they first got whiff of the sterile, hospital aroma that came home with him on his clothes and belongings. Earth, mud, grass, stagnant water and fox poo being more to their liking.

Looking back, I recognise that Monty and Totty were our glue ... they were close to us and they kept us all closer to each other. When Ollie was in hospital, they were what kept the rest of us sane and functioning, the warm, reassuring hugs that wrapped around each individual: they sat with us, walked and ran with us, and they simply gave themselves to all of us when that emotional bomb dropped on our family in the summer of 2008.

I felt that we had been on some kind of conveyor belt of treatment. You can wish for it to run fast or a bit slower, but it will always take its own route and pace. No two routes are the same, despite identical diagnoses, and as parents we want to help, but once we realise that the treatment path is outside our control, we have to take each hour as it comes in the rough periods and each day as it becomes smoother. Our children are snatched from their healthy lives and put on that virtual conveyor belt. All we can do is trust that we will be able to lift them off at the end. We must wait, hope, trust the medical team and be there for our child whatever the outcome.

Having Ollie home meant that it was time to make plans and it was thanks to the charity Make-A-Wish that we were able to take Ollie on his trip of a lifetime to the Give Kids the World (GKTW) resort in Florida. After all his time in hospital wired to machines and the rigours of chemotherapy, Ollie was bursting to get over to the States and experience fun and freedom again. Harry too was excited to be going on holiday and have his family all back together. I guess they were bursting to go anywhere after all that they had both been through, but this place was so special. Spread over almost one hundred acres of land, the resort offers parents with children with life-threatening or life-limiting illnesses the chance to holiday together and enjoy a range of activities, every one of them geared to having fun safely. Families, just like us, from all over the globe, gather there to relax together, a world away from the restrictions of hospitals and monitors, for a week of just being themselves but with all the support they may need discretely at hand. Going to GKTW was truly a wish come true for Ollie, for all of us.

Before we set off, I could never have imagined how magical and life-changing that time away would be for our family, and for me.

We hit Florida in July 2009 and arrived with the boys, having been treated like mini celebrities. Ollie and Harry were invited up to the flight deck before the plane took off and the flight crew made sure we had everything so that we could relax and enjoy this special trip that was happening for us.

The excitement of the journey overtook every bit of the anxiety that came with the lead-up to our trip. It was such a relief to see a huge sign saying *Give Kids the World Welcomes Ollie Uglow* being held up as we walked out of the baggage hall and into Arrivals. I could feel the muscles in my face stretch with happiness as our 'greeter', the lovely Phil Cooper, stepped forward to intercept us. Phil, a retired police officer from the UK, and his wife Jo, a retired dental nurse, were part of the volunteer workforce at GKTW who made everything so perfect for our stay. The couple settled in Florida and decided to donate their time and skills as members of the team of 'Angels' – that's what they call the volunteers at Give Kids the World – and truly lived up to their name. The passion Phil and Jo offer to their volunteer role comes from a deep place and their kindness is tear-jerkingly inspirational.

While Ollie, Harry and Mike were enjoying the supervised activities with the other parents and children, I found myself drawn to the volunteer services department at GKTW. There, I felt the meeting of empathy and selflessness reach down into me in a way that I didn't expect and had never experienced before. Something clicked inside me. I reminded myself that I was a guest parent on holiday with their child and likely to be looking at all of this through a pair of rose-tinted spectacles. I needed to appreciate that I was a parent who, not so long ago, had been released from the pressures of a hospital inpatient nightmare, so holidaying in Florida was bound to be the best holiday EVER! The thing is, it really was the best holiday ever and it came at exactly the right time. I'm absolutely convinced that I was meant to meet Phil and Jo.

The Cambridge English Dictionary's definition of volunteer is: 'A person who does something, especially helping other people, willingly and without being forced or paid to do it', but that says nothing of the special qualities an individual must have to be totally present for someone else, for someone who is vulnerable. Being an Angel is hard work but our lovely new friends displayed the unwritten skill in the role – they made it look easy.

My brain was ticking over the whole time we were there. Thanks to Phil and Jo, I had found something in me to tap into that I didn't even know was there and I blame them entirely for planting the volunteering seed in my brain.

Before we left the resort, I promised our Angels that I would be back – as a volunteer. To keep me connected to the place and to my promise I took a photo on my phone which I have looked at many times since, especially when I've needed a jolt of energy or inspiration from my Florida mentors. The photo is of the motto written at the entrance to one of the pool complexes. In my opinion, it is one of Winston Churchill's finest: '*We make a living by what we get but we make a life by what we give.*'

I decided to carry that motto with me, in my head and in my heart.

8

Our growing family

HOME LIFE AND EVERYTHING THAT WENT WITH IT just kept going full-speed ahead from the moment we touched back down in the UK. My small business was busy and we still had hospital appointments and check-ups to attend with Ollie, who was looking and feeling so much better. He was getting stronger by the day and that made it all the more difficult to accept that it would still be two years before he could be given the all-clear. We have a little saying in our house – KBO (nice people say ... Keep Battling On!). It's another inspirational motto from our victorious WWII Prime Minister that's so perfect for the Uglows battling against the invisible enemy that seemed, at last, to be on the run. That particular enemy had cruelly barged its way into our lives and so we knew that we would forever be looking over our shoulders.

Like swans, working hard to display an air of serenity on the surface, we were paddling like crazy beneath the waterline and, believe me, it's an image that's not easy to maintain. Despite the fact that they had daily needs that added to my workload, once again the dogs glued us all together. I'm pretty sure that's where I got the idea that if two dogs had helped us to get this far, more dogs had to be a good idea. Don't they say, be careful what you wish for?

In September 2010, Totty gave birth to ten beautiful, golden puppies: seven girls and three boys. It was a home birth and first to pop into the world was little Jessie, who we later decided to keep to join our growing golden clan. Totty was a wonderful earthmother who doted on her brood, gathering them into her to feed, never leaving anyone out of the busy and never-ending lick-and-wash round, and happy to show off her family to the rest of us and anyone else who came to coo over her and her babies. There she was, my running partner ... a new mother!

I'd never had any intention of being more than a one-dog owner, never mind the owner of two golden retrievers and there I was with a litter of ten pups, which was not only planned but very much wanted.

I'd hoped that Totty would pass all the necessary Kennel Club health checks needed to give her the all-clear to become a mother – and my wish had come true. From that moment, with everyone watching and special friends waiting for a pup, including Sarah and Patrick, who years before had placed Monty with us, the pressure was on me to get it right. It was both exhausting and exciting as we waited for the litter to arrive.

Totty had been totally relaxed throughout the entire nine weeks of her pregnancy, leaving me with my head deep in the pages of *Book of the Bitch* and *Breeding Dogs for Dummies* (yes, they are genuine book titles), which I frantically covered in scribbly notes to answer my many questions or raise points to cover over the phone with Totty's breeder Sarah or our mentor Catherine in France, who both kindly and patiently offered their extra guidance. I was excited, anxious, terrified and proud of myself all at the same time! What was I doing? Maybe I just needed to know that I could do it?

The puppies were a real joy to have around. Yes, it was extra work for me but that didn't matter, it wasn't what it was all about. Maybe the puppies were another time-guzzling distraction from Ollie's unresolved situation or something that, in some part, I could control. I was at the centre of it all and the dogs never failed to give me their attention, gratitude, companionship, a listening ear ... and hairy love. I thrived on the extra role of looking after the litter 24/7. It was also a great way to fundraise and give back to the charities who had supported us. Payment for each of the pups went to the charities who had supported us, and that included a donation to GKTW.

Monty was being a big brother about things, sniffing around as if asking if he could help Totty with her mothering or the little ones' playing. Of course, he also loved the fact that there was lots of extra food being prepared for Totty while she fed the ten hungry mouths. Harry and Ollie were delighted to have puppies in the house and even happier knowing that Jessie was going to be staying with us, to be a part of our family. I had half-thought that Jessie could be Ollie's puppy and be his golden companion as Totty had grown so close to Harry in past months, but Jessie only had eyes for Mike. Perhaps as he delivered her, the first pup of the litter, that is why. We went from two dogs to twelve and then down to three once the other nine pups left for their very special new homes. It was great fun, but of course at times, in reality, it was absolute organised chaos!

Before the puppies left, they had become a busy entity of their own and everyone who heard about them wanted to meet them or, at least, see pictures. It was in this whirl of puppy stardom that I had agreed to a photocall with the children's cancer charity CLIC Sargent as part of the pre-publicity for the 2011 London Marathon. I had run the same event for this charity in 2009 and it had become very dear to our hearts. I knew the value of all the wonderful social workers and counsellors who had supported us through Ollie's time in hospital and wanted to make the best of a brilliant chance to raise awareness and funds for the charity.

We had photographs of the puppies taken and post-cards created as fundraisers. And in a moment of sheer madness, I agreed to a media photocall with all ten puppies. I don't know what I was thinking! It was their biggest opportunity to showcase how gorgeous they could be; they did that while I confirmed why it is rarely a great idea to attempt a line-up of bouncy puppies who all want to skip away in different directions in a photo studio! Totty gazed proudly over her brood but clearly had no control over them whatsoever. They were a team of free spirits and it was up to me, with the help of a hefty supply of dog treats and a couple of willing volunteers, to get them organised.

It was Jessie's first PR event and we were treated to a lovely glimpse into the developing ways of this little whirlwind. Even as a pup she was a solid, round thing with big paws and had all the makings of the dog I now describe as a huge personality with a 'floofy' coat. A born entertainer, Jessie has always had a sparkle in her eyes and loves to be busy. She is the one with the big retriever instincts who circles and looks everywhere until she can find something to present as a gift. She always insists on giving gifts to house guests, even if it is their own car keys! The time she 'lifted' my friend's astronomically expensive Louis Vuitton shoulder bag from the hall and delivered it to her in the garden. I held my breath as I saw Jessie trotting towards us. To compensate for her short legs and the bag's long handles, my clever dog tilted her head back so the bag didn't drag on the ground! Unless you're quick to head her off at the pass, Jessie is happy to help with the online shopping delivery too, by retrieving it bag by bag and redelivering it to you in instalments! Jessie, the busy little body who loves home and makes servants of us all. Her confidence was there from day one, along with her endless capacity to make me smile.

Running two more London Marathons – this time for children's cancer charities CLIC Sargent and then Teenage Cancer Trust – after Ollie had been treated, had been important to me and I planned to do another, but at the same time I recognised that it was unfair to ask the same friends and family members to sponsor me. I had to come up with something new to give back. But the real focus for the rest of 2010 and 2011 had to be reaching the date for

Ollie's all-clear. The oncologist said December, hopefully before Christmas. If all went well, this meant an all-clear forty months since his diagnosis. The better Ollie was doing and the nearer we got to Christmas, the more I wanted to book a family holiday to take everyone to ski in the mountains to celebrate. But I had to ask myself: was I tempting fate?

Life had chucked us a curveball as it does everyone from time to time and for now we were managing to keep leukaemia at arm's length. Like most parents of a child undergoing long-term healthcare issues, in and out of hospital, it feels as though someone has grabbed your child from you and thrown them, like a stone into a deep puddle, and you're caught in the ripples. We would all take the illness from our child but we are never given that option. It leaves you feeling that there's no accounting for what fate will deal you next, and for me, that meant keeping the demons on the run for longer. We booked the holiday in the Alps and crossed every finger and toe that we would be able to make it a celebration.

A year after we decided to keep Jessie, Catherine called from France. There was a new litter on the way and there was a puppy for me ... if it was the right time. Goodness me, of course it was! Little did I know that the puppy, yet to be born, was the one that would change the course of my life.

We first met Leo and the rest of his litter at two days old. We were dropping Monty, Totty and Jessie off to stay with Catherine and Sven at their home in France en route to our holiday in the Alps to celebrate the all-clear Ollie had been given when he saw his consultant on 21 December. The sight of the litter of puppies in their home added a super-special touch to the start of our trip.

We watched them being fed by their beautiful mother Mimi and fell in love with all of them right away, so it really didn't matter which one of the boys Catherine decided was the right personality for us. Their dad was there, too, Rayleas Just a Joker ... the entertainer of the household who had just the most perfect name. He practically introduced himself and I often see the same gentle 'how lovely to meet you' trait in Leo when he introduces himself to a new patient. I wanted another boy because we had Monty and our two gorgeous girls, Totty and her daughter Jessie. I liked the idea of having two of each and if I am honest, my relationship with Monty had become so deep over the previous few years, I wanted to ensure that he passed on all he knew on how to look after me while he was young enough to do so. That probably makes no sense to someone who doesn't own a dog but I suspect that it will resonate pretty strongly with those who do.

We settled on the name Leo as a family, while relaxing and eating lunch together outside one of our favourite restaurants in Les Arcs. From that first meeting, the pup we named Leo became our link with happy times and positive new beginnings.

By the time we called back into Catherine's seven days later, we had skied and talked about little other than the puppies and this time we were able to hold them. Sadly,

Ollie was sporting a broken collarbone, which was the only downside of our lovely trip away, but it didn't stop him cradling all the pups – and one of them was going to be our Leo.

Leo stayed with Catherine and her family until he was 16 weeks old and had his pet passport, which allowed us to bring him into the UK. It was April 2012 when Mike and I drove to France to collect Leo with Ollie while Harry was staying with some schoolfriends. As soon as I walked into the house, I saw our large new bundle of golden love cradled in the arms of Catherine's daughter, Emilie. The second I committed to taking a pup from this litter I heaped a load of hope on this new boy bringing light and perhaps luck into our lives. As Emilie passed him into my arms, he snuggled into me and I'm sure I saw the first glimpse of that now-familiar Leo aura. Catherine told me that this one was very laid-back and chilled and I felt immediately that this pup was special. Just holding him gave me a feeling of ... hope.

As we prepared to leave, Leo was passed around for a last cuddle from the family. Jonathan, Catherine's son, said how emotional it was saying goodbye to this one as he had been a lovely pup to have around. For me, it was a giant relief that I could take him home with me.

As we travelled through France, Leo was slightly unsure about being on the move, but we soon worked out that as long as Ollie kept his hand in the travel crate, our pup was reassured, calm and quiet. But when we arrived at the Channel Tunnel, Leo was ready for a welcome cuddle break and to be fussed over by officials checking his pet passport.

Leo was probably only too glad to be out of the car even if it was just for a short time before we had to continue with the journey. But the calm only lasted until we swapped to driving on the left! Leo was a French dog and used to French ways and the camber of French roads, so no wonder he felt sick and whimpered in protest. To him, we were driving on the 'wrong' side!

By the time we reached Hampshire and home, Leo was fast asleep and snoring. As the car slowed and pulled up on the drive, his eyes started to open and I heard the little yawn as he stretched out his legs then slowly wriggled up onto his feet. His canine family were all waggy-tailed and excited to see him and Harry was there too. We introduced Leo to Monty, Totty and Jessie and it was a joy to see our laid-back boy accepted immediately into the pack. The others showed him where the dog room was and the route out of the dog flap. A quick plod out of the back door for a pee and soon he was stretched out in front of the cooker, his chosen spot, as if he had been living there for weeks. I noticed how much he liked to lie there, looking at us all. It seemed to me that he was observing the hierarchy of both the human and canine family he had just joined. Sometimes Jessie rocked up to see if she could tempt him away to play. She bowed down in front of him, using the full canine body language to say: 'Come on, don't just lie there, you lazy lump ... let's play!' The two of them then started to play like pups do, a bit of play, a tug on an ear, maybe a bit of pretend bitey face, and then concluded it with a turn away at the end of playtime so Leo could return to snoozing before the next play session or meal.

They became the best of friends and with just a fifteen-month age gap they enjoyed a close bond right from the start.

Leo is Leo with both his human and canine family. As a puppy, and to this day, he ritually presents himself to whoever he finds in whichever room he plods into and then sits or lies beside them, offering himself for attention. He just loves being touched and he is the king of the 'leaners'. Monty was a good introduction to a dog who likes to 'lean' but when Leo arrived we realised that Monty was a mere amateur! Leo has a way of adding pressure the longer he stays with you. If you sit on the floor with him, it won't be long before he's not just beside you – if he can be, he's all over your lap!

When he was old enough, Leo added hugging to his repertoire. And I don't mean the annoying 'jumping' at you kind of hugs: I mean a full-on paws-around-your waist-hug, which he makes special by gently pressing his feet in as if to squeeze you. The thing with Leo is, he doesn't jump up, he levitates, so his actions, even for a big dog, are very gentle. When the others do it there is a 'bounce' and they seem to land on you, but with Leo, he just arrives in front of you with feet ready to go around you! I have one of his lovely hugs first thing every morning when I go down to the kitchen to let them out. He stands there offering his hug for as long as I want to receive it. Then, when the others come close to me, he finds a way to get between them if he decides that I should have his attention more than theirs. Ideally, with Leo, you need an extra hand so you can always have a hand free to touch him the whole time he is near you. If you stop and take your hand away, he looks sad and disappointed and then nudges into you to start again. A true needy-nudger!

It seemed to me that from the moment Leo joined us he brought joy and light and the good things carried on happening. Harry, inspired by his brother's recovery, decided he wanted to row the English Channel solo in aid of Make-A-Wish. In completing it in August 2012, he set the record as the youngest person to complete this challenge and raised almost £20,000 for the charity. A feat that happily resulted in Harry meeting Olympian Matthew Pinsent at Henley and thereafter being recruited to the junior development squad at the Leander Club in Henley. I was so proud of him, I could have burst. Two summers later, in 2014, he took the silver medal at the Coupe de la Jeunesse in France for the GB junior team. All that from the boy who just wanted to try out rowing, to see if he liked it better than rugby. If she could speak, I think Totty would have been so proud of her buddy too.

Things were going well at last, and to be honest, apart from accompanying Ollie for his annual follow-up appointments, I never wanted to see the inside of Southampton Children's Hospital again. All the incredible staff who looked after him would forever be special to me, to all of us. Mike still worked there, but I had done with that place for now. At least that's what I kept telling myself. The thing is, what I did next didn't quite fit the intention.

The deal that I made with myself on the hospital stairs in the twilight hours continued to haunt me. I had a deep sense that I needed to give something back to the hospital that had given Ollie back to us. It had to be something extraordinary to repay such a debt, so I trusted in the hand of fate to deliver the answer.

Part Two:

Dogs Working Miracles

9

Get a dog!

WHAT, FOR ME, STARTED AS A WAY of giving something back to Southampton Children's Hospital was to become a huge and incredible part of my life. I just didn't know it at the time. All I knew was that I had to give something back. And when I get a strong feeling like that, it's like an itch that has to be scratched.

I was on a routine shopping trip to our local Sainsbury's in Hedge End when I noticed a couple of volunteers doing an in-store collection for the charity Pets As Therapy (PAT). My eyes were drawn to the dogs, so I stopped for a chat to find out what they were all about. It was odd really because I must have seen them there before but maybe been in too much of a rush or too distracted to linger. But that day was different.

There's something universally lovely about people who love dogs and I experienced this right away with the PAT community. I've no doubt at all that I came over to them as a bit of a whirlwind of enthusiasm and determination to extract all the information available on how my dogs could join the ranks of these yellow-kerchief-wearing heroes.

Jennifer at head office probably thought a tornado had hit town, especially with all my questions!

Not twelve months after that first meeting with the volunteers at Sainsbury's, I had all four of my dogs qualified. What the volunteers had shared with me was dynamite. My 'itch' was scratched and now it was metamorphosing. From that day on, I was in no doubt at all that my dogs had what it takes personality-wise to make the grade. And that's the key to Animal Assisted Intervention – the animal has to have the perfect temperament and enjoy what they are doing to be able to support sick and therefore vulnerable people.

I started low-key with visits to a local residential care home with Monty and, later, eased Leo into visiting this new environment with all its different smells and the new experience of visiting lots of elderly people. He was a young dog but no less able to give the residents what they loved, which was simply a visit from a kind-hearted canine.

There was one thing about visiting older people that I hadn't considered – some elderly residents instantly pat a dog rather than stroke it and Leo wasn't quite so keen on that approach; it just makes him cower and blink a lot. I should have known better as my own father was a dog 'patter' and that's just the way he was and I had noticed that most of my dogs didn't always like it. Being aware was enough to solve the problem and so Monty, the happy plodder, was the dog most suited for this role. Totty, the sassy outdoors girl, was fine too, but she wasn't likely to stick with much beyond the meet-and-greet bit before moving on to the next person, which worked fine too as we met the residents together in the day room. After visiting for a while, I realised that some people were happy with Totty's style of visiting while others didn't mind a longer, lingering experience with Monty; Leo as the 'junior' member of my little team was kept in reserve.

Every resident has their story and as I discovered, very often there's a dog in there somewhere. A few months after we started, I was asked by the matron to visit one of the residents who had become withdrawn due to her dementia. I didn't see why not – after all, that's the wonder of dogs, they treat everyone the same. My grandfather had suffered from dementia and I thought of him as I walked to this lady's room, remembering the agonising confusion that he had struggled with during that phase of his life. The visit didn't get off to a great start.

'Would you like to see the nice lady with her dog?'

'Who are you? And what do you want?' came the reply from the elderly woman wearing a double-string of pearls and quite a stern expression.

Despite the gentle introduction from one of the care staff, this resident was the toughest audience Monty and I had encountered in our short visiting career so far. I stepped forward and as I did, Monty padded a little closer to our new friend, who suddenly had plenty to say.

'You're always late,' she said brusquely. 'You had better go and grab your cup of tea because my daughter will be home soon. I wonder what kind of homework she'll have. It's Wednesday so she will bring the food that she cooked in her home economics class ... unless it was good then she will have eaten it on the way home! And it will be maths homework today, which she won't want to do. Oh, she is so hopeless!'

As I listened, the lady held out her long, bony hand to take Monty's lead, so I offered her the middle bit while I kept a firm hold of the handle. Meanwhile, my dog sat quite happily at her feet. I must have looked a tad confused.

I had no idea what our new, very elegantly-dressed friend was really talking about but while all this was happening, I noticed a photograph in a brass frame, dusted and positioned in pride of place along with a small collection of more recent colour shots of people I assumed to be her relatives or friends. The sepia shot showed a younger version of the woman I was visiting, with her own golden retriever by her side. I guessed that was the image from times past that sparked the idea for our visit. For just a few minutes it seemed Monty had been the bridge between this patient's past and the present. His presence had helped unlock a portal into her memory, helped her make a very vivid connection with her daughter, her dog and Wednesday afternoons over fifty years ago.

It was such a powerful event to witness, like being held under a spell cast purely by Monty's presence. And Monty? Well, he was just enjoying her attention.

It took a few minutes for the care assistant to encourage the resident to loosen her grip on Monty's lead, but once she did, the spell was broken. I reported back to the matron what had happened and asked if the lady did have a daughter who visited her. And if she did then would she like me to take Monty in when she next visited because I wanted her to see her mother talking so animatedly about the old days. Sadly, that meeting wasn't possible, but she did have a daughter who confirmed to the carers that everything her mother, a retired headmistress, had shared with me was true: the dog, the school, Wednesday's cooking class and the dreaded maths homework. I felt privileged that such a precious memory had been revisited through my appearance with Monty.

I couldn't help but wonder what was going on? Such powerful connections don't happen through mere coincidence, do they? It seemed to me that Monty unlocked memories so strong that the lady holding his lead was virtually transported back in time. This was a wonderful revelation to me and it moved me to thinking how powerful a therapy dog visit could be. Were dogs really able to be a bridge for dementia patients?

'Get a dog!' That was one of the bright ideas that came my way when the last thing I needed as a mother who had just started a small business, and whose husband was working beyond full-time was that, but there was something in the idea that had me thinking. Dogs have always held a special and positive place in my life and most dog-related memories take me to a happy place of laughter and beautiful, warm, fuzzy recollections of genuine companionship.

My childhood was spent on Dorset's coast. Of course, I didn't appreciate it then but later I could see how having the beaches of the Solent, such a beautiful playground, so close by, must have influenced my love for the great outdoors and the joy of feeling the wind on my face. Mum, who was a teacher and ran a nursery school, and

Dad, a lecturer at Bournemouth College, which is now Bournemouth University, were dog lovers, so thanks to them my younger brother, Kieran, and I had the company of Nini the corgi. I was only nine when Nini passed away but when the old photographs come out of the boxes at home, I'm met with a selection of images of a very young me, laughing away with a plump and smiley corgi at my feet.

Kieran and I had guinea pigs for a while but when they died, they were not replaced, and then poor Candy the cat was only with us about twelve weeks before we lost her in a road traffic accident. I imagine that was when my parents decided against having any more pets. Losing them was just too traumatic. I feel sad that I can't recall Nini's character very well, but I do remember her company and her comfort in our pretty normal 1970s upbringing.

The local comprehensive school gave me an OK grounding and I excelled in the subjects I loved, but no one could inspire me to love the sciences that I found tough. Maybe if my brain had been wired that way, I would have followed what had become something of a family tradition to become a teacher, or pursued a career allied to medicine or maybe even veterinary medicine. I had considered physiotherapy for a while but of course that required science too, so was probably out of reach. Anyway, not long into my A-levels I decided to kick academia into touch and find a job instead.

Soon I was working for Barclays International at the bank's head office staff department in Poole. The job fed my independent streak as I travelled the fifty minutes there and back every day to work and was part of a team supporting staff in far-off places around the globe, including some, like Vanuatu, that I had never even heard of. It was all very exciting for someone who had just left the confines of education, but, when the offices relocated to London, I chose to move on and ultimately ended up working in a private hospital in Bournemouth as part of the administration team. I started there just before I was nineteen and it wasn't that long before I was able to buy a small flat.

I loved the role and the increasing responsibility that the hospital's owners entrusted to me including the introduction of a new (it *was* the 1980s) 'state-of-the-art' computer system. I worked hard but thrived on everything about that job: the lovely people, the place and the camaraderie, everything because I felt I had found my niche in a healthcare environment. In time, I also moved into admin management and took on the role of personal assistant to the owners and that meant I sometimes spent time working at their home as well as the hospital. Working for them gave me a great buzz and there was something else I loved about that job – the family had the most amazing dogs.

Duke, the white German shepherd, was their guard dog, so his sheer size and ferocity was enough to scare folk away and, at first, that included me! He had a bark that put the fear of God into anyone who approached the property and when he added his 'all hair and teeth' glare no one was going to risk getting in his way. Duke was a snarling tyrant ... and also a smiling pussycat! When he got to know the sound of my car and clocked that I was welcomed into his owners' home, he decided that I must be a friend of the family, so he was wasting his time giving me his full-on scary guard dog act. I saw him in action a few times when the odd delivery guy decided to risk tiptoeing past him and, believe me, they didn't do it a second time! Duke was no thug; he was a very loyal and intelligent dog who knew when to put on and take off his work 'face'.

Memories of Duke are very vivid but I think that's because he made such a big impression on me as a larger-than-life character in every way. I had never met a dog like him before, but the family's pet dog, Roddy, found his way directly to my heart, I think because he reminded me of a childhood friend's dog. Roddy was a golden retriever with the most incredible big head, dark eyes and gorgeously handsome expression. He had been involved in a freak accident as a youngster, landing badly after leaping a garden wall. His injury left him a bit wobbly, so he was always more than happy to spend hours pottering around at home or snoozing in front of the fire.

When I first met Mike, we used to walk Duke down to the beach some evenings and I always looked forward to seeing lovely old Roddy on our return. Although he couldn't move too briskly, he managed to find his super-powers when treats were on offer! That was a goldie who had a nose for the biscuit tin and put snoozing top of his priority list. He had such a loving personality and whatever Roddy did, he did it in the style of a fine old gentleman and, without doubt, sewed the golden seed in my heart.

Despite all the great warm memories of dogs past, I was still ignoring the inner voice, which was now a loud whisper telling me how much a dog could fill the 'gap' in my life. I was running out of delaying tactics but then I thought ... Let's try hamsters! The boys thought they were fun, but in reality, they were a couple of brilliant, furry escapologists who had us ripping out kitchen plinths on several occasions trying to find them. I wondered if I was feeling how my parents felt – that pet ownership wasn't supposed to be that stressful!

In 2003, with the hamsters slowly driving me mad, I found myself in a local shop looking at a card pinned to the notice board. The handwritten card read: 'Golden retriever puppies for sale'. I decided I would take the number down and phone when I got home. Excitedly, I told Mike when he came home from work and eventually after a bit of persistence, he agreed we should go and have a look at the weekend. We arrived at the address and parked in a side road only to hear lots of dogs barking and see a side gate with a sign on it that read: 'BEWARE OF THE DOG S#!T'.

Ignoring that, we approached the front door and could hear little yaps of puppies. The door opened straight into the front room and there were two litters of golden retriever pups, pee and poo everywhere, very few toys and a disgraceful mess that absolutely stank. We chatted briefly with the lady at the house, who told us we needed to pay a deposit to secure one that day, but we made our excuses and left. As we left, both the boys in the back of the car were in floods of tears wondering why, when the lady said we could definitely have one, there wasn't a puppy for us! Safe to say that Mike was not convinced he wanted a dog after that. We didn't know a thing about puppy farms then but we knew enough to know that a good breeder would not have a room full of puppies skidding along the lino in pee and poo. It was foul! I felt deflated but knew it was for the best. I had wanted a dog for so long, it just had to be right.

10

Hello, Monty ...

THE NEXT FEW WEEKS PASSED and as I felt that we were getting over our ghastly puppy farm experience I popped into the local vets to see if they knew of any golden retriever breeders. Eventually someone passed on a number but all the puppies had been reserved, so I was relieved that I hadn't said a word to the boys. I didn't want to raise their hopes again.

I decided to leave my 'get a dog' project a while. Life picked up pace again and Mike certainly wasn't rushing to have a dog. He was concerned that we probably had enough on our plates. But then, sadly his father was diagnosed with cancer at the age of seventy-three.

Mike had examined his dad when he visited his parents at home in Gloucester. Feeling the lumps, he knew that it was not going to be good news. It took a month for the full diagnosis to be made and the doctors identified that it was an inoperable disseminated cancer and that he was dying. The harsh acceptance of this was a massive wake-up call for us both and although we had said many times that life was not a dress rehearsal, here was the starkest reminder that if you have a desire to do something in life, you have to get on with it, *carpe diem*.

My father-in-law's rapid decline was the catalyst for my call to the Kennel Club. A very helpful lady gave me details of Catherine Zingg who, she said, was both an international judge of golden retrievers as well as a breeder and at that time lived little more than an hour away from us. I only wanted a pet so was not really looking to talk to an international judge! Never mind, I made the call and explained that I was looking for a puppy. After answering what seemed like a barrage of quite searching questions about us and our home circumstances she gave me the number for Sarah, who had a litter due. 'Well, you can come and see me if you like but I cannot promise anything will be available,' said Sarah. She was holding her cards close to her chest!

A few days later we were on her doorstep and I was reminding the boys not to touch anything and to be on their best behaviour as this house had puppies inside! As we got out of the car it just felt different – not at all like our last experience. The adult dogs greeted us as we stepped through the door and Sarah was soon firing questions before taking us through to the whelping pen in the kitchen. There, was a beautiful litter of three-week-old puppies being fed by their mother. One by one, Ollie and Harry held the pups, and then Mike and I. It was incredible – somewhere in that litter was our puppy. We asked for a little boy, but it would be a while before we found out which one Sarah had chosen for us and we could take him home. Even so, I felt massively relieved and, to be honest, I think I was more excited than the children!

We had planned to go away that October half-term but we had a very short time to get used to the shadow of terminal illness hanging over our family. It was a difficult time for all of us, especially Mike who was working his way through a sticky pit of emotions. On the one hand he felt he needed the break from his busy work schedule, on the other he needed to be around for his mum and dad. It was a no-brainer – we cancelled the holiday.

We had to think of keeping Harry and Ollie's spirits up, so on the first Saturday of half-term I took them to see the pups and on the way we chatted excitedly about what we could do instead of going away on holiday. We had seen the litter twice but still hadn't met our puppy, so I was hoping this time would be it. The thing is, I had squashed this visit in ten days ahead of when I was due to collect him, which originally was planned to be after our holiday and once the boys were safely back to school. Never mind, it would cheer up the boys and I couldn't wait to see the golden bundles.

When we arrived, I wondered why one of the gorgeous chunky puppies was wearing a bow – and then Sarah picked him up: 'Lyndsey, your family has had such an awful time lately, I think you should take him now. It will give you all something to enjoy over half-term.' I tried not to cry and gabbled on about how I had not expected this and so didn't have the money with me as it was only a visit ... but I could see it didn't matter to Sarah. She was smiling at the boys cradling their new playmate.

As we carried him to the car, I was hit by all the practicals: I had planned on spending half-term buying a dog bed, bowls and all the equipment our new recruit needed. But I wasn't going to worry about that. By then I was 35 and I wasn't going to wait any longer for my first golden retriever! Besides, Sarah was insistent: 'Don't worry, Lyndsey, we know you, take him now and send the balance. I will be in touch anyway, wanting to know how my baby is, so I'll be on the phone later and tomorrow and the day after that!'

I remember having tears in my eyes as we left with our puppy in a wicker basket on a towel, plus a bag of food, lots of puppy paperwork and a few poo bags. The boys stroked him all the way home, where we surprised Mike, who had arrived home from work and wasn't expecting to meet Monty ... our new puppy!

Seeing the boys fussing over their new companion was magical and Monty took it in his gentle stride. It took some time to persuade Harry and Ollie to go to bed and leave Mike and I to get to know our golden baby. Watching Mike, the man who for a long time was not keen on getting a dog, hugging our tiny puppy was incredibly emotional for me. There was this six-foot-six man experiencing what I now know to be the power of the human-animal bond.

The next day Mike returned to be at his father's bedside and for the next few days he was backwards and forwards to Gloucestershire at all hours of day and night trying to be there for his parents and yet also be there for his patients at the hospital. And so it went on until one of his colleagues, who is a close friend, saw how exhausted he was and told him to stop coming to work and focus on his dad.

Monty arrived just a couple of weeks before Mike lost his father and all of us felt the comfort of that little puppy's affection. Mike found himself enthralled by this new addition. He hadn't been brought up with dogs and had no experience of them apart from accompanying me on walks with Duke early in our relationship. For all of us, I truly believe that Monty was the most unifying member of our household at that difficult time.

Monty's laid-back personality gently eased us into dog ownership. All we really knew about keeping dogs was based on time spent with Duke and the golden oldie, Roddy. But all that added up to was knowing something about older dogs, not the bouncy puppy kind, so having Monty's patient and forgiving ways was an absolute blessing. He was what we now think of as a typical retriever – meaning that he was a real food monster! He quickly worked out that keeping an eye on the boys as they carried their toast to the kitchen table was well worthwhile. If he gave one of them a nudge to the back or side of the knee, the toast slipped off their melamine plates and there was Monty, available to helpfully clear up the spoils! Even when the boys used a thumb to clamp their toast to their plates, he adapted his ways: he sat statue-like by the table for the duration of the meal, eyes full of hope, with a single drip of drool extending slowly from his lips to his chest.

Early mornings were Monty's favourite time. We have always been early risers in our family because Mike was always out of the house well before 7.30am and I was out with the boys on the school run by 7.50. Monty liked to nip from the kitchen out into his run before bursting back through the dog flap ready for his breakfast and then enjoy follow-up snuggles with the boys and the prospect of a sneaky snack. After the school drop-off, I took him to the beach or the local country park for our special time together before heading back home, where I worked on my small business, which was then based at home, and all the usual work of a mum. Sometimes a friend joined us on the walk but most times it was just the two of us for our 'me and Monty time'. He was the apple of my eye.

A loyal and biddable dog grew from that little Monty puppy. I could not have asked for more from him. He came to me at a time when I felt that something was missing from my life and dark thoughts were circling, and he brought the sunshine with him. He was friendly with everyone and everyone wanted to spend time with him. He was fun and by that I mean he was a minor criminal: he stole food from the work surfaces in a way that only a puppy with inexperienced owners can. He chewed up the boys' toys, so they soon learnt to put them away, and he trashed the occasional shoe if anyone was stupid enough to leave one lying around. His most accomplished role was as destroyer of dog beds! Eight cheap beds were completely destroyed until we decided to invest in an Orvis memory foam one, which proved to be utterly Monty-proof because he clearly found it so comfortable it was worth keeping in one piece.

He even helped us in ways that he could never have known. When our finances were low, we moved him on to food from our local cash and carry and he uttered not a word of complaint. It was so lucky that Monty had an iron constitution because we had to chop and change his food every few months for a couple of years, based on the best bargains around, and his gut just accepted it all. Of course, we now know it should have been a slow transition off one food and on to something new. We were so lucky to have him as our first dog as he forgave our ignorance in so many ways.

Monty was happy as long as his family were around him and he had me in his sights. Even when his eyes were closed and he appeared to be asleep, Monty always sensed when I was going to leave the room. I can imagine him thinking: 'Nip to the loo on your own ... Now why would you want to do that, boss, when I can come with you?'

For a very passive dog, Monty never liked to miss any action. We thought our garden was dog-proof but he soon proved us wrong. Getting the whiff of our neighbour's Old English sheepdog who was in season, Monty found a way to nip out to introduce himself. On another occasion, when we thought he had excused himself to take a nap on his bed in the kitchen, we discovered that he had escaped through the dog flap, gone through a gap he had found under the garden fence and taken himself for a run across the golf course! These were just two of several late nights when Mike, who was the orthopaedic surgeon on-call, joined me in the dead of night, torch in hand, to coax Monty home. When eventually he returned from his midnight romp, we sleepily ignored his very muddy legs and went to bed! At least Mike managed to get a few hours' rest before he had to be up to do the morning ward round.

Very handsome and really golden, Monty attracted lots of attention on walks. One time, when the boys were with their grandparents giving Mike and I an opportunity for a walk on our own, we took Monty along the prom at Bournemouth and were stopped in our tracks by a retired golden retriever judge who was extremely interested in his breeding. She loved his look and said that he was one of the old types and had such a wonderful colour. I thanked her but wondered what she was talking about. All we could say was that we bought him from a lovely breeder in Sussex and that her friend in Surrey had his dad. I don't think we sounded clued-up enough for this lady, who had such an eye for Monty and really was after his pedigree lines, but she nevertheless suggested that we consider showing him. The more she praised Monty, the prouder we became. We thanked her and walked away like clucky parents of an over-achieving child! But we did have a laugh about showing him. Mike had come a long way in agreeing to have a dog in the first place; he was loving having Monty around but I could never see us showing or breeding from him. Apart from experiencing a serious surge of pride we never gave it another thought.

11
Along came Totty!

IN 2007 I WAS RUNNING FOR MY SANITY and as time went on my running increased and so did Monty's. Yes, I was training for my first London Marathon attempt, but it was the running and the time alone with Monty that was holding me together. My loyal friend had already seen me through some tough times. As I've shared with you earlier, our walks and runs helped me organise my feelings. There were days when I dropped my sons at school and the fog in my mind only lifted once I started walking with Monty. I was still anxious to make sure that I put up my shield at the school gate and hopefully, had been all smiles so the other parents didn't pick up that I was really struggling.

Harry and Ollie loved school, Mike had a great job and we were all a happy family, but the initial dip in my mental health after our return from Australia in 2000 was there again and still taking its toll all these years later. It didn't help that my little business was in trouble and I was spun back into questioning myself and my ability to trust my own decisions and my faith in others. What was wrong with me?

All the jigsaw pieces were thrown back in the air. I know there is never a time limit on these things – we can wish the dark thoughts to disappear at some point – but, inside, we know that's not possible without some help. Seeing a counsellor was proving a good move for me. I had to admit that I couldn't do this alone and I was lucky, I had Mike, my rock. But if there was one 'person' who knew everything there was to know about our lives and my feelings at the time, it was Monty.

Monty ran with me, walked with me when my energy was low, or just sat with me; whatever we were doing, I was talking to him. Sometimes we decided to have a change from the country park and the beach by heading off to the New Forest, where we walked and I talked, walked and then we walked some more. Once I parked the car and Monty had completed his ritual big sniff and obligatory first pee, we were on an adventure together. I felt free in a way I didn't anywhere else back then and I was able to unravel things stored in the tight pack of thoughts in my head.

Out with Monty, I was in control of my thoughts with no distractions or responsibilities to hold me back. Monty was beside me so all was fine. I always felt safe with him chugging along at my side. He was one of those solid, dependable types who make you feel that everything is going to be alright, even if you don't believe it yourself. When I looked at Monty, I saw someone I trusted with my life and by just being there he reassured me that my trust was not misplaced.

I remember one of our New Forest adventures, back in the days before Google Maps on mobile phones, we walked for over an hour but, clearly, I hadn't taken a necessary 180-degree turn, so the car park I returned to was not the one in which I'd left my car. As soon as the realisation hit me, I imploded into a tearful shaking mass, convinced that we were lost and that I'd never make it out of the wilderness in time to collect the boys from school. Monty didn't flinch! He didn't move from my side and happily engaged with the people who came to our rescue. They were locals, which was handy as they were able to point me in the right direction for the car that was parked near a pub I could name and, as it happens, I wasn't far away from it. In my moment of dire panic and complete overwhelm I was convinced that we were lost and that, of course, it was all my fault. There ... not good enough to even walk my dog and make it back to the car without messing it up. That was in my head, but Monty knew different and I think our rescuers saw that in him. It was Monty who stayed calm and helped me by staying close – my constant support and my keeper of secrets.

It was in August 2007, the summer after my first London Marathon, that Totty arrived in our home. She came from Sarah, the same breeder as Monty, and having her with us felt perfect from the start. We were now golden retriever crazy! Totty, even at eight weeks old, was so very different to Monty. Yes, she was a puppy and this time a girl, but, as I've already said, she was also a complete and utter whirlwind! I never guessed that it could be so much fun having two dogs in the family and I'm sure Monty felt the same. He went from being my shadow to experiencing a degree of divided loyalties: part of him regressed to 'big puppy' stage and an almost guilty expression of: 'OMG, boss, this pup is so much fun. I love you, boss, but do you mind if I share some of my attention with her?'

Seeing Monty and Totty bounding around together was incredible! They clearly adored each other and we were loving having them living with us. As Totty grew, we noticed that she wasn't just the storm to Monty's calm: she was her own independent, self-contained little being. She loved being outdoors to the point of preferring to lie quietly outside by the back door on the cold patio slabs to any of the comfier options of relaxing in her bed in the kitchen or leaning her head in someone's lap.

At times I wondered if she really liked living with us because she didn't show any desire to glue herself to my side, but then, Monty had secured that spot long before Totty appeared on the scene. Maybe that's why she directed her adoration towards Mike. It was lovely to see him get a slice of the action as Totty used to get so excited when he came home from work that she could hardly contain herself. Within two seconds of being inside the front door, Mike was covered in blonde canine hair and being offered a toy! He was loving having two dogs – thank goodness!

Looks-wise Totty displayed the finer features of a female retriever and the most amazing tail, which I watched grow beautifully, and it never grew straggly like some do. Back then, I didn't groom my own dogs but somehow she never looked scruffy or shaggy like Monty always did between his six-monthly grooms. These days I can barely resist tweaking their coats every couple of weeks, but back then owning two dogs made me want to learn a bit more about trimming them and so I asked the lady at the groomers to show me the basics of grooming, doing their ears, necks and nails. And at the same time, I discovered something very peaceful and therapeutic to enjoy with Monty and Totty.

Totty had a lovely personality. To me she was like a sweet friend who never gave us any trouble, but she was someone I admired for her spirit and her fearlessness. While poor Monty had wide eyes, ears pinned back in panic whenever he heard a loud noise or, horror of horror, fireworks, Totty just carried on regardless. Nothing phased that girl and her love of the outdoors was a joy to watch because she really smiled when she was romping about in grass or water and she never failed to make the best of the last sunbeams in the garden for a nap. Her slim, taut body gave her a beautiful line in the water and as a leaner, smaller version of the athletic Monty, once she was old enough she was a good running partner, eager and focused as we jogged along.

I still haven't had a better running partner than Totty. Her pace was perfectly in sync with mine and sometimes, maybe twice a week, when she was old enough, I made sure that it was just the two of us so we could get a proper run together. She would cast a glance up to me to make sure we were both enjoying it.

Our second family pet fitted in perfectly and by the middle of 2008, life was great. I was running now with two dogs, both of whom were loving it as much as me, and we were back to the more normal distances after my first marathon. I thought I had another marathon in me but I was also well aware that it would be hard to juggle all the activities that the boys were into plus the longer-distance training that I needed to make time for. Life married to Mike was great but his job had to come first, so he was hardly ever around until after the boys' bedtime and his on-call rota meant he needed to be at the hospital some weekends too.

I admit that there were times when I felt lonely but there were so many more positives coming into the mix then: I was more in control of the shadows that had lurked over me and the strength and confidence gained from the marathon run the previous year was still with me. I did that for me ... and I needed it. I proved to myself that I was still inside this body, I could control me and what I wanted for myself. Monty was such a big part of helping me achieve that and ultimately Totty became such a big part of my future running. I was making things happen, feeling good and life was on the up.

My little home business was starting to make money again and that meant the business debts could be paid and with that came a massive element of relief. It was my mini venture and only meant to be an additional income stream, not a pain or a source of worry for me. It was my thing and besides, Mike had enough on his plate with his work; the last thing I wanted was to give him any cause for concern. He worried about me, I knew that, and he knew when it wasn't going well. Some of the big corporate people letting me down in this venture hurt me in a deeper way than the financial loss. Getting back from that was like getting to know myself all over again: maybe I needed to be less naïve, less trusting, more aware of others' agendas?

I told the dogs all about it and I always felt that Monty listened to every word. I didn't expect him to have the answers but I felt that he had my back and that I could say anything to him and he'd be fine with it and love me all the same. Not only did he hear me but I didn't have to hold anything back. I could be totally honest with him and not be criticised or judged. I felt stupid enough, so I didn't need anyone else to echo it. My dogs' constant care for me was everything.

I learnt a great deal in the process of getting my business back on track and that was as much about trust, human nature and people in general as the world of business. We decided to celebrate by ordering the new kitchen that we'd been promising ourselves for years. I watched the project come together and with each piece that moved into place I thought about what had been achieved and sacrificed along the way and what it represented: we had survived a near business disaster that had clipped my confidence – but I had put that in the past. Things were getting better. The new kitchen had been completed and it was time to go on holiday, but was it *tempting* fate to remove the labels from the new cabinets? I left them on, just in case.

Three days after we returned home from our holiday, we received Ollie's diagnosis.

12
Pets As Therapy

MONTY WAS MY FIRST THERAPY DOG and he saved me in so many ways. Little did I realise how much I would depend on him again when Ollie was so ill. Only the survivors get to record history and it was survival that made us stronger than ever as a family.

When I first started to take the dogs into local care homes around Southampton, I was probably a little bit naïve in my desire to share the love and companionship that I had with my dogs with others. All I know is that it made me feel good and after all, my dogs had personally helped me over the line with Ollie's leukaemia. If I could help just one more person feel better through my dogs then I was on my way to paying back what I felt I owed for Ollie's recovery. I could never have imagined how this initial 'feel-good' feeling of mine would develop, although the clues were right there in front of me from the start.

Walking into the day room of a care home with a dog must for them be something like walking onto the stage to face an enthusiastic audience – minus the applause but with all the wide-eyed adoration before you. They approach their new fans with a slightly quizzical expression, possibly wondering which one of the outstretched hands will reach them first. I've seen people take small children in to visit elderly relatives and the effect is very similar – a tidal wave of love and affection from the residents and an initial look of fear and panic from the children! I've no doubt that it can be quite intimidating for a child to be met with a gallery of faces and loud 'cooing', but I can only say that my dogs took the same response in their stride. I've a notion that it was the appearance of the cups of tea and lashings of Rich Tea biscuits that boosted their interest.

From the moment we stepped into the day room the dynamics changed – and that wasn't one care home, it was all of them. The smiles, the reaching hands and the animated chattering. I know we were only seeing the residents who chose to be there for our visit, but I felt that we were making connections in some way and on some level with every touch and stroke that came our way.

Joan, one of our first care home residents, loved seeing Monty and Totty so much that every goodbye was one huge emotional pull. Our visits became a real highlight in Joan's life in the home and for me it was an absolute pleasure to share my dogs with her. Her smile made it all worthwhile and reminded me why I was there. Of course, Joan had no idea of the reason that drove me to volunteer with my dogs or how much she gave to me in every visit.

She directed her conversation through whichever dog was with me and who sat patiently soaking up the fuss and attention for as long as it was on offer, but when Joan finally had to give up her grip on their thick, golden coat,

I became aware of the hold she had on my hand, which was just as strong. One day, as her thin, twig-like fingers of more bone than flesh gripped me, I felt such a deep sense of longing from her that I had to gulp back the tears. We connected in that moment and I understood her desperate loneliness – I had been there too and I felt it again without a single word being spoken.

I felt almost guilty that I had to leave her, but having been there a while visiting as many patients as I had, I knew I had to get home. I also knew that there had to be more to this than just visiting elderly people with my nice dogs. Something was taking place in that moment of connection – in all the smiles in the room, the eagerness to embrace my dogs, Joan's grip on my hand, I really felt that we were creating some kind of bridge between us. For the person running her hands through the dogs' golden coat the connection was whatever they wanted it to be: a treasured memory, to feed a basic need for affection, to feel wanted again or even just a warm response from another living creature. To just feel something ...

I took a leap of faith and the next time I went into my volunteer admin job on the ward where Ollie had been treated, decided to talk to Kim Sutton, the head of voluntary services at University Southampton Hospital NHS Foundation Trust (UHS). I asked if they ever had Pets As Therapy (PAT) dogs visiting and to my delight, she told me they did. I completed the forms, had hospital environment assessments of the dogs completed by Kim and a few weeks later, we started visiting the adult wards of Southampton General too – first with Monty to see how things went and then over the course of the next eight months, one by one, all the dogs had a hospital assessment.

Taking the 'girls' in for hospital visits was a bit of an adventure. I wondered if outdoor-girl Totty would take to it at all but she was fine and everyone loved her. A few weeks later, I took Jessie, who was in her element; Miss Floofy coat was born an entertainer, more accurately a comedienne, as she has an endless capacity to make me smile. But, as a born-at-home, live-at-home pup she has only ever seen her human family as her 'staff'! She always gives the impression that she allows us her company just in case she needs something – and that 'something' is usually food! It drives her every waking thought. Although she is far more ladylike than the others as she doesn't drool, she certainly knows where to position herself for any handing out of treats.

When we go to walk off-lead in the country park in the morning, she always walks behind me. I'm not sure if this is down to nature or nurture, but I suspect nurture. She was 'dog number three', so when out walking on the lead it was Monty on the outside, Totty on the inside and Jessie closest to me, but sometimes I asked her to walk behind me and that's where she picked up a handy hint. From behind she could see my hand go into my pocket for treats. So, when she's off the lead, she keeps a keen eye on my hand and if she sees it going in, she will pull in parallel ... just in case there's a biscuit on offer! Jessie is a foodie opportunist, cheeky, bouncy with a highly active body that likes to keep on the go, which made her hospital assessment day a little challenging.

Leo's first trip to the hospital gave me no cause for worry whatsoever. I had an inkling he would be fine. He had, after all, qualified when I hadn't even anticipated he would. I had booked the PAT dog assessment for Monty but Leo was along for the ride as I didn't want to leave him at home with the girls. He was only nine months old and I thought this visit would be great for socialisation from the safety of his pop-up crate. The assessment was based around the outside of a library and a day centre for adults with special needs and although this was unfamiliar ground for Monty, he was happy being with plenty of people, some in wheel-chairs, who were keen to fuss him and just might have a snack about their person. He stayed his cool and calm self as the assessor ran through his checklist. Monty ticked all the boxes: he walked to heel, allowed the assessor to touch all over his body and be groomed easily without protest, and finally, he showed absolutely no aggression when approached by other dogs. Once we had passed all of the outdoor exercises, he trotted inside to see who I could introduce him to.

It was at this point that, as agreed with the assessor, I went back to the car to collect Leo and the pop-up crate so that he could watch Monty in action even if he wasn't allowed to join in. I didn't want him to be out of my sight nor miss the fun on a day out.

Monty was introduced to two young guys who loved dogs and one by one they started fussing over him, but it soon became obvious that they were reluctant to share him. Sensing this situation could turn awkward, I asked the carers if we could do one at a time and maybe see the second guy, who was now standing with one of the carers about three metres away, holding his hand out waiting his turn. On the assessor's suggestion, with Monty's assessment now complete, I swapped the dogs so Leo took his turn out of the crate and Monty went in – much to his disgust! As the guy who had been so patient stroked Leo, he smiled and bent down to gently hug the very calm, happy puppy close to him – and would not let go! It was one of those sweaty 'what do I do now?' moments but I had no need to worry at all. Leo was literally laid-back, leaning in and enjoying being hugged.

What happened next was amazing too. The assessor, clearly impressed by Leo's sweet-natured performance, said: 'You know I can assess Leo today too, if you want me to. He is just old enough and from what I've seen, he's a natural.' I couldn't believe my ears. Brilliant! 'He has already helped himself with the "meeting a stranger" test,' he went on. All you need to do is let me complete the other parts of the assessment and see you walk him and that should be fine.' Just in case he had a change of heart, I quickly transferred Monty back to the car and ran Leo through his paces for the outside assessment with Monty watching his little protégé from the boot. And that, as they say, was that.

Monty and Leo passed the assessment in November 2012, earning the right to wear the yellow PAT dog kerchief, and all the charity then had to do was obtain references about me. By May 2013 Jessie and Totty were listed, too. I had started my route into Animal Assisted Intervention (AAI); I just didn't know it was called that then. But seeing Leo enrolled confirmed something for me – just what an incredibly biddable, calm dog I had on my hands. He'd been exactly who he needed to be with that vulnerable young man at the day centre who simply wanted to hold him and be comforted. In retrospect, it was a massive sign, a huge indication that Leo was a true therapy dog-in-waiting.

Catherine had chosen him to be our puppy because of his special personality. In the four months he stayed with her in France before he could come to the UK, Leo showed all the traits of being a placid little chap who was bound to fit in with our team back home: Monty the loyal guardian, Totty the sassy outdoor girl, and Jessie the independent whirlwind. She was right, we needed a little bit of calm in our lives. And after nine years as a golden retriever owner at that point, I thought I had seen most aspects of the breed's personality variations – that was until Leo arrived.

As you are aware by now, laid-back is always the first description of Leo that comes to mind. Mike occasionally calls him 'Tim Nice-But-Dim', after the character played by Harry Enfield on *The Fast Show* in the 1990s, and, if I'm honest, Leo can appear a bit dim at times. However, I like to think of him as considered, more a deep, sensitive character who doesn't necessarily have to always 'do' mainstream retriever things.

For one thing, he has never been destructive, apart from refashioning the zip on a very expensive Dubarry boot. But as Catherine says, 'It is never the dog, always the owner', so that was my fault for leaving it to dry in the dog room right next to his bed. Another unusual trait for a retriever is that Leo doesn't have an insatiable appetite. Snacks have never bothered him because his drive is for a cuddle or a tennis ball reward and this has been his way from puppyhood. His slow eating worried me so much that I decided to supervise him at mealtimes while keeping an eye on the other three who were hovering over him, eagerly waiting for him to take his last mouthful so they could move in to mop up his leftovers. I stayed with this routine until I convinced myself that his speed had picked up enough for me not to worry and I could return to dishing up the dogs' food and go into the kitchen next-door to clear up after breakfast.

Eventually, Leo appeared with his tennis ball looking incredibly pleased with himself, leaving the others to lick microscopic morsels of food off the edges of the bowls before bounding off into the garden. I accepted his gift of a toy or a tennis ball and congratulated him for being such a good boy for eating up all his food. That clean bowl deserved lots of fuss as I felt so relieved to see it. After a couple of weeks, I took them all for a routine vet check and it was noted that Jessie was heavier than she should be, while Leo could do with a bit more flesh as he was getting very 'ribby'. I was shocked! I had to put that right so I gave him more food. A few weeks later I took him back to check if my plan was working. Nope! What was going on?

I had to get sneaky with my detective work, so I set up my iPad to record the next mealtime and then sat down to watch the results. Shock, horror! All four dogs started together, heads down in their own bowls ... Jessie finished first, way ahead of the others. No surprise there, the greedy monkey! Then, she picks up a tennis ball and drops it by Leo's bowl. He can't resist a ball so he turns, picks it up and wanders into the kitchen to give it to me. And guess who finished off his food? Jessie had secretly trained Leo to give up half of his dinner! Leo, not being a foodie, was quite happy with the arrangement, especially as he ended up getting loads of fuss from me, which is what he ultimately prefers!

This adorable but occasionally daft, very special, exceptionally kind dog of mine was, I felt, in my care for a reason. And I knew what that reason could be – it was all to do with the special way Leo connected with people.

The visits to the general wards at the hospital were going well, so I was taking a dog into the hospital once a week and then doing a fortnightly visit with one of the others to the two care homes. This gave me two volunteer stints every week: one at the hospital and one in a care home. I loved both but I really loved visiting the hospital.

Some of the characters we saw in the elderly care unit made me chuckle. The ladies there were in a bay of six and it wasn't unusual for those who were awake to gossip about the ones who were asleep and I got to hear all about it while my dog was being fussed! The dog heard it all and I said nothing!

The men's elderly care ward was entertaining in a different way, but then I didn't always help myself. One day, I stood at the entrance of the bay of patients and said in a bit of a loud voice: 'Good afternoon, gentlemen, would anyone like to stroke a dog?' If only I could have taken the words

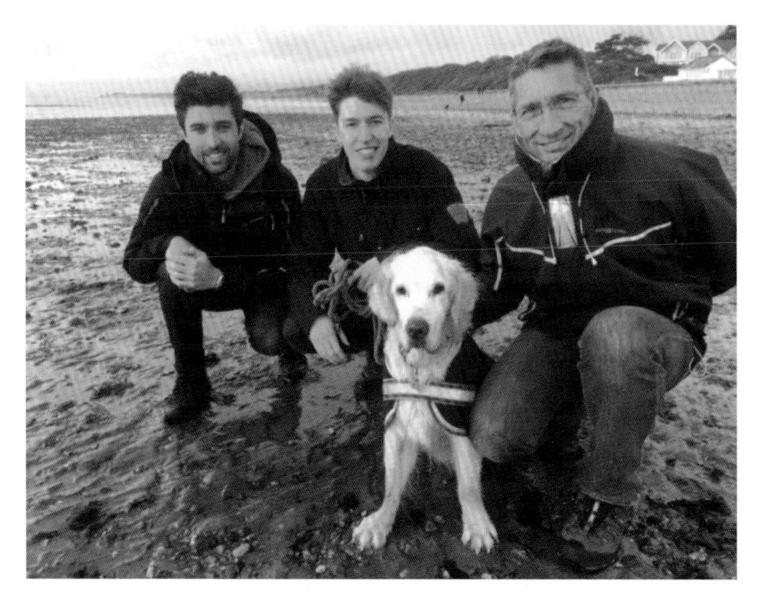

Harry, Ollie and Mike with our first dog Monty, who was then aged 15 years.

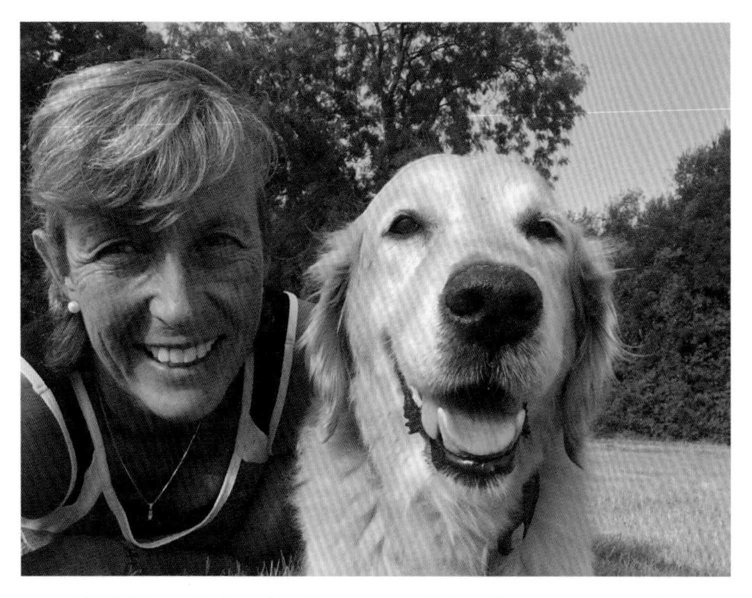

With Totty during the time some of the villagers apparently called me 'the running dog lady'!

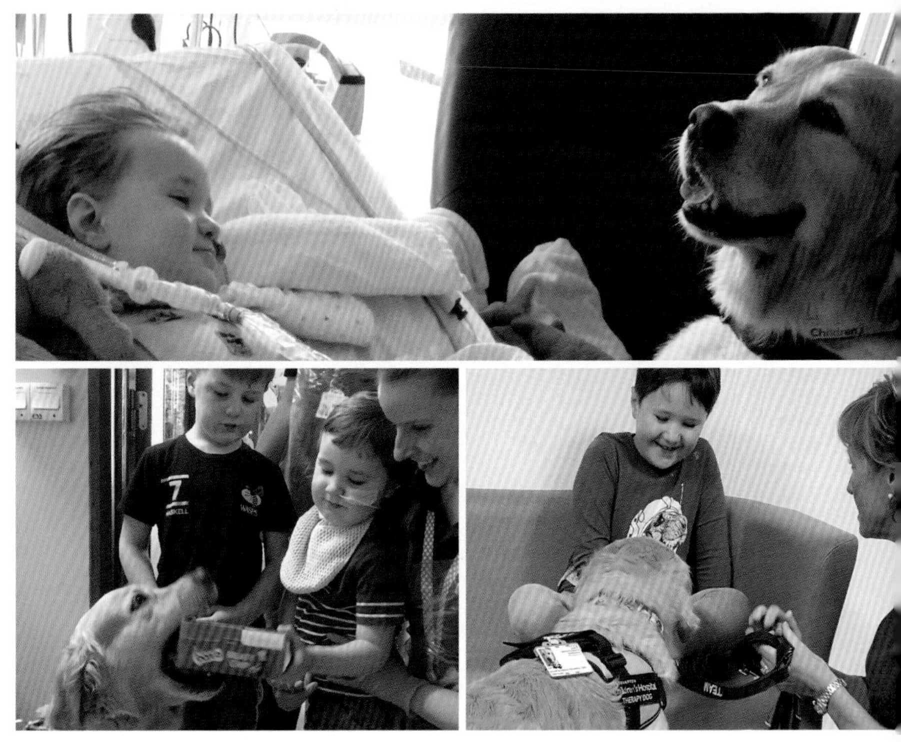

Oscar the patient, who smiled when he saw Leo in intensive care. His parents later described it in a television interview as a miracle.

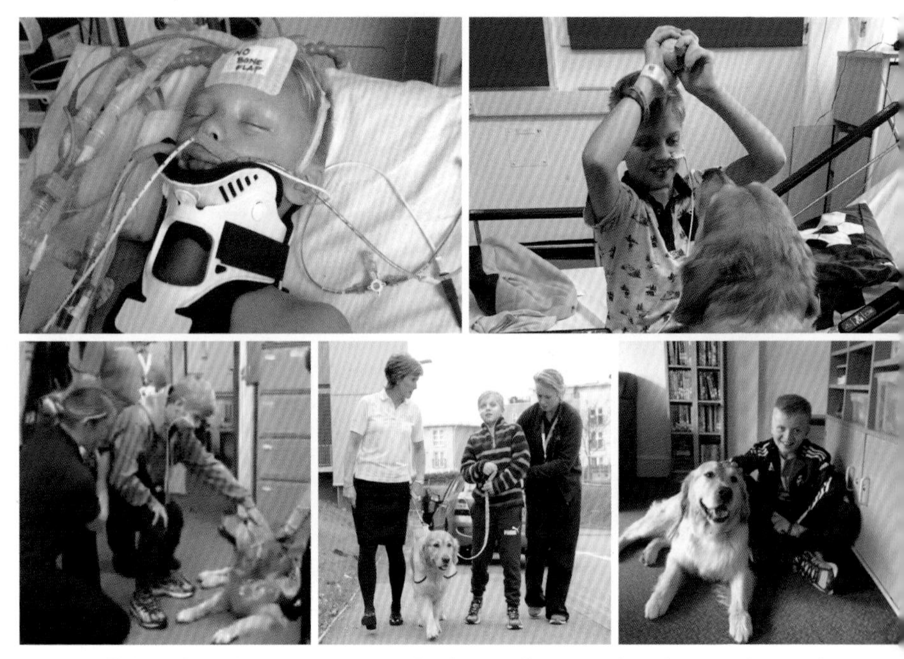

Felix – from intensive care to discharge after months of expert hospital care, interspersed with some great times with the therapy dogs.

THE DOGS CREATE A FUN BRIDGE BETWEEN THE PATIENT AND THE HEALTHCARE ENVIRONMENT.

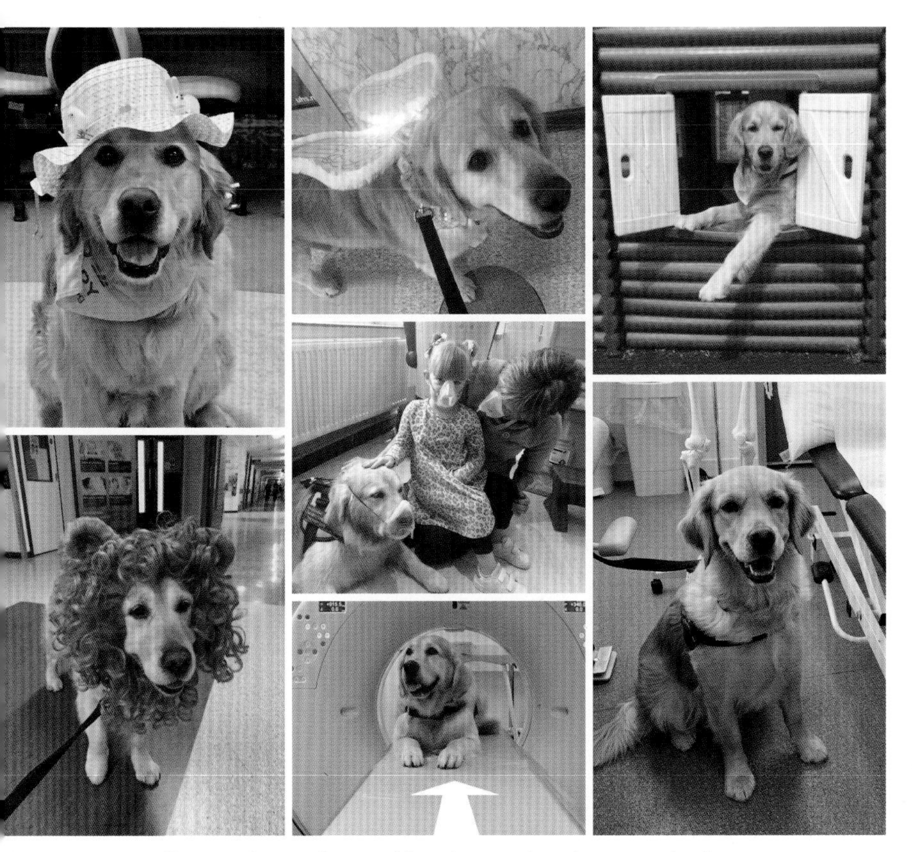

Centre picture: Leo and I make wearing the anaesthetic mask into a role play game for Lillian.

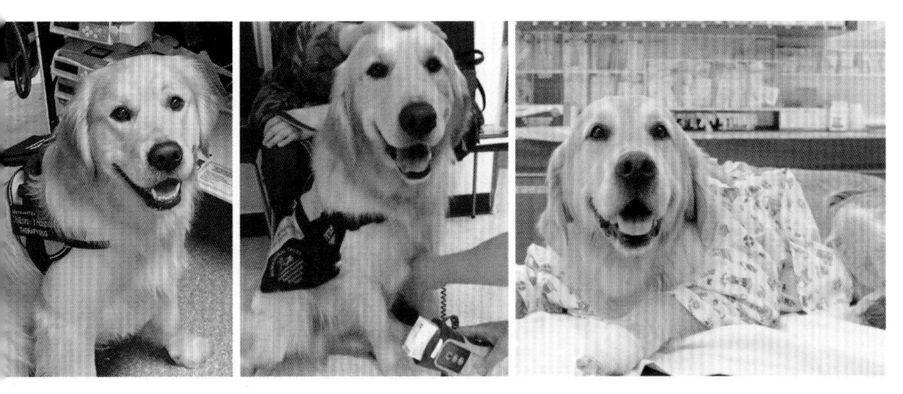

More fun. Quinn sits with the PICU patient retrieval kit, Archie shows the children how easy the pre-operative tests are and Leo shows them how to wear a surgical gown and relax on the trolley in the anaesthetic room.

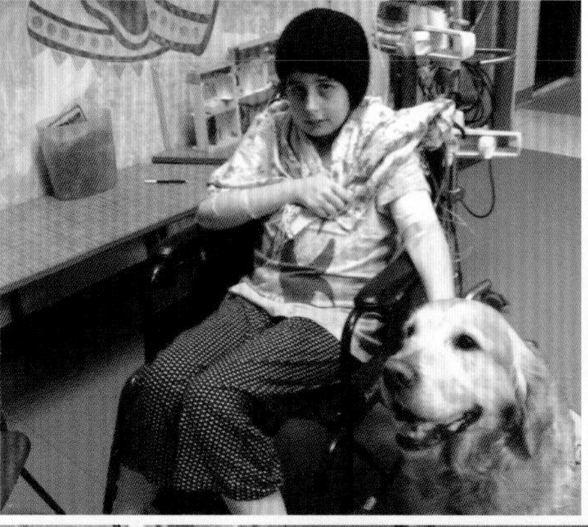

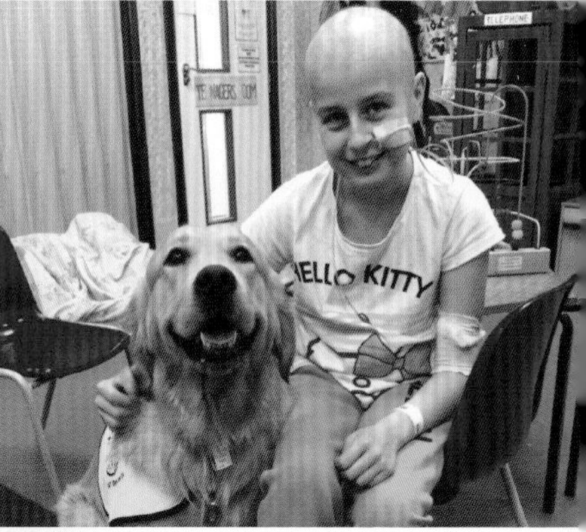

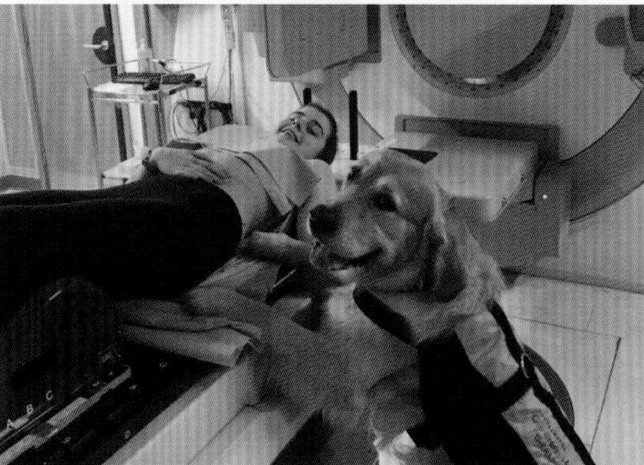

Above and left: Alice – lots of canine cuddles and AAI support helped her four year cancer journey.

Below: Archie – paralysed and in paediatric intensive care, his monitors showed his vital signs improved when Leo visited.

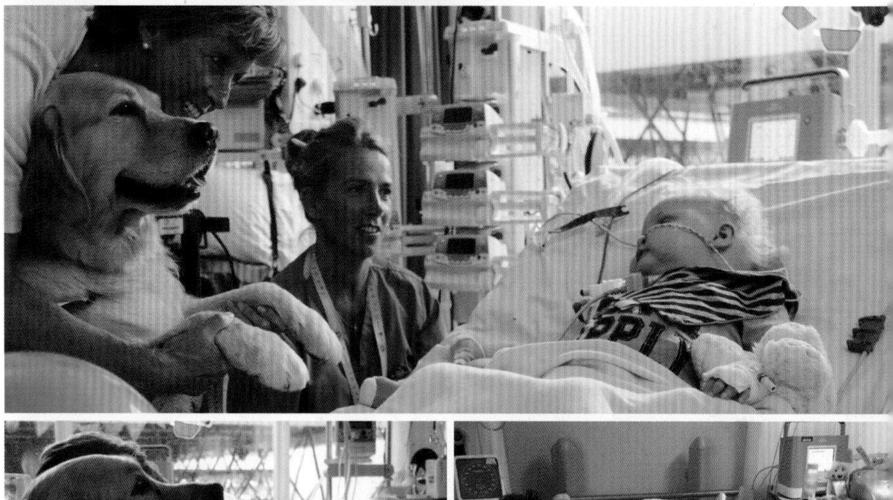

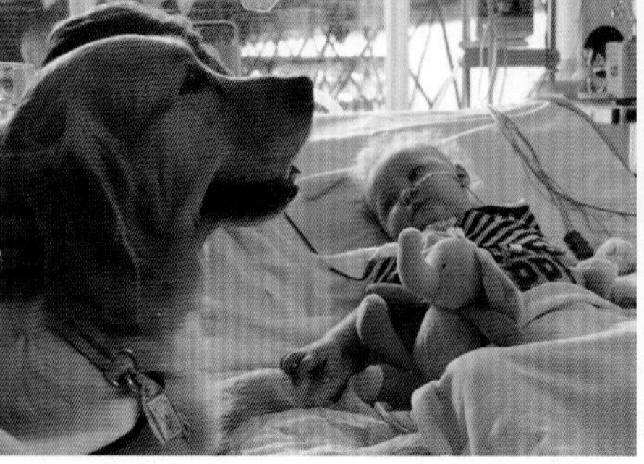

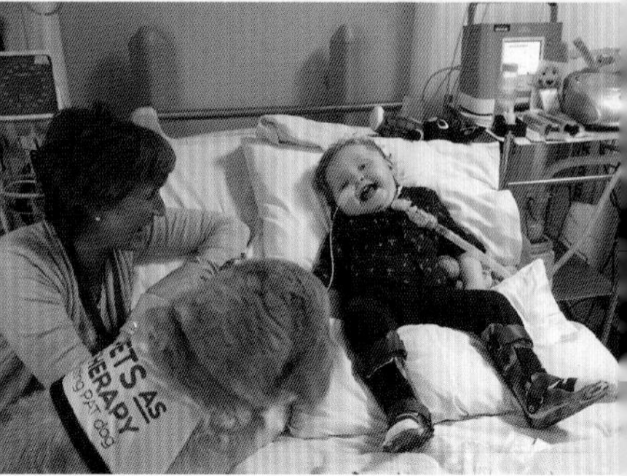

AND MANY, MANY MORE . . .

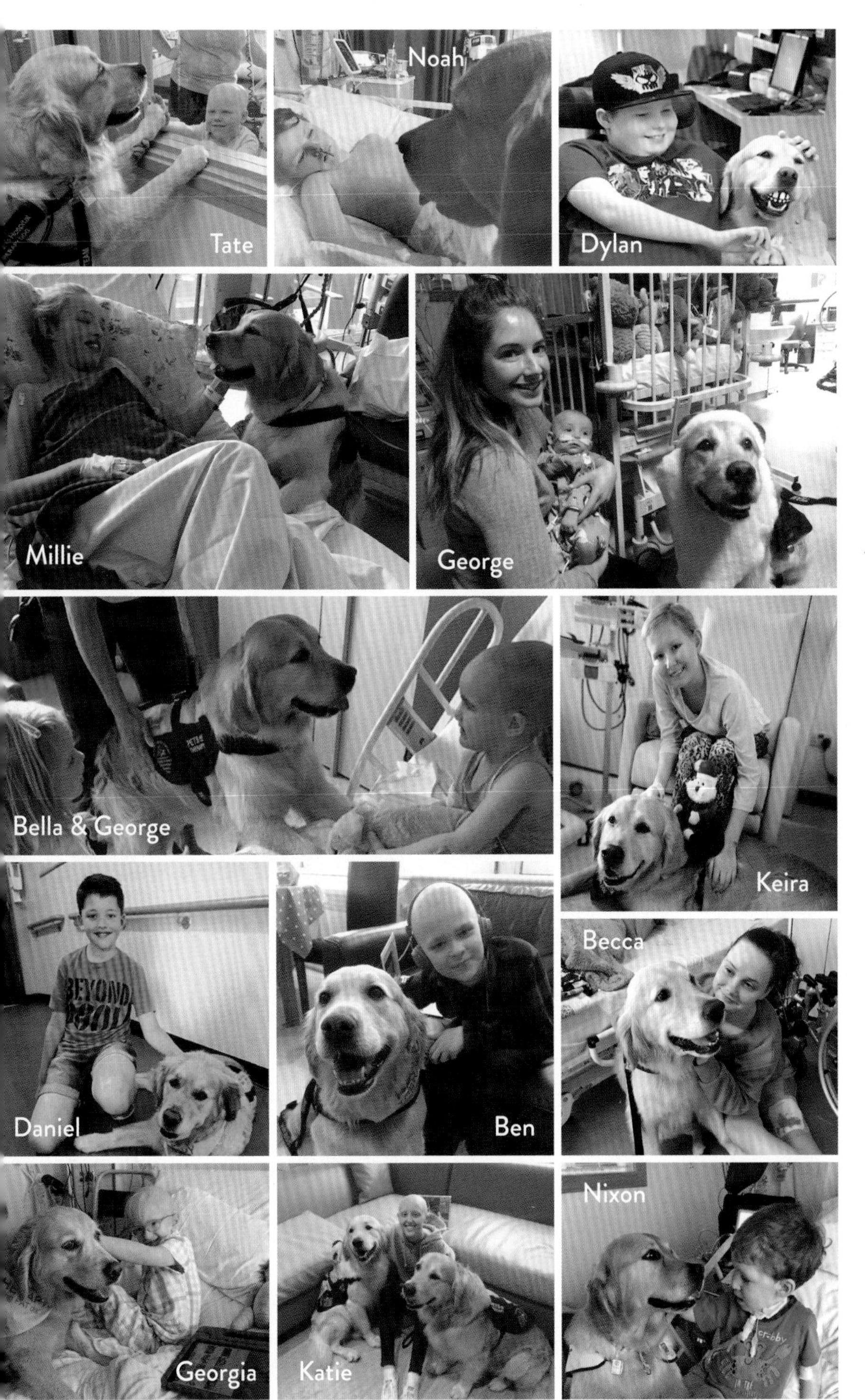

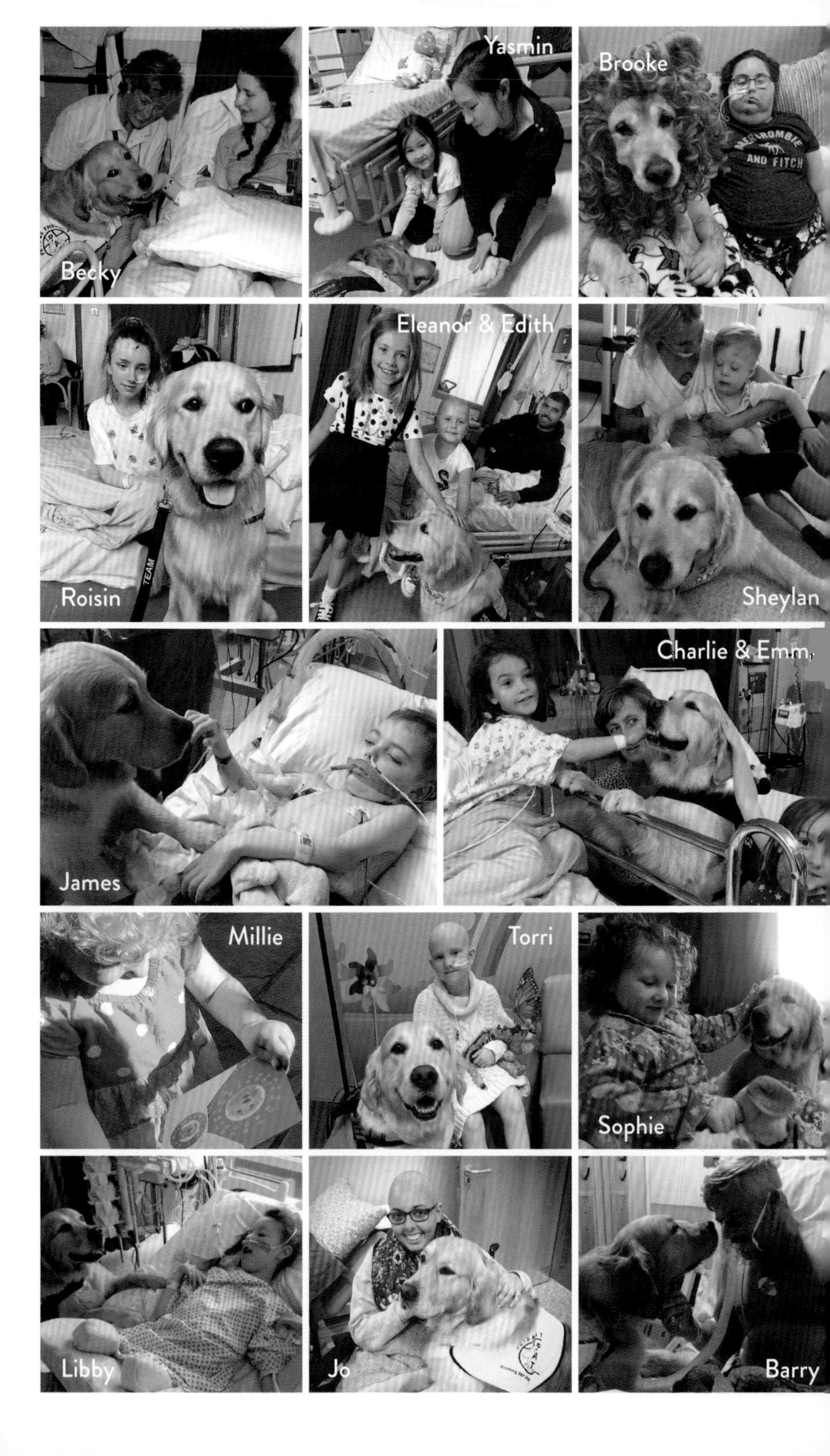
Becky
Yasmin
Brooke
AND FITCH
Roisin
TEAM
Eleanor & Edith
Sheylan
James
Charlie & Emm
Millie
Torri
Sophie
Libby
Jo
Barry

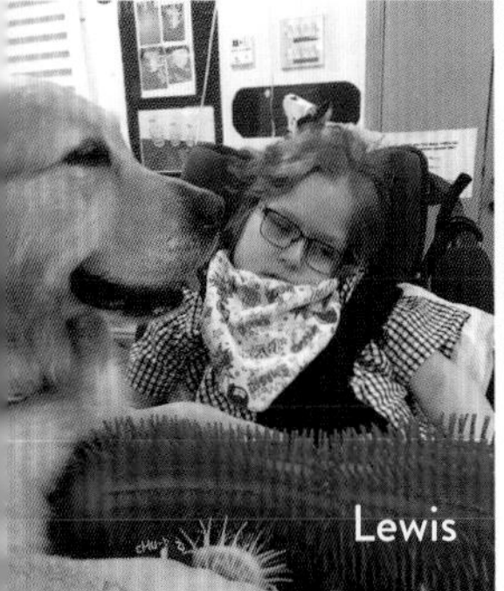
Lewis

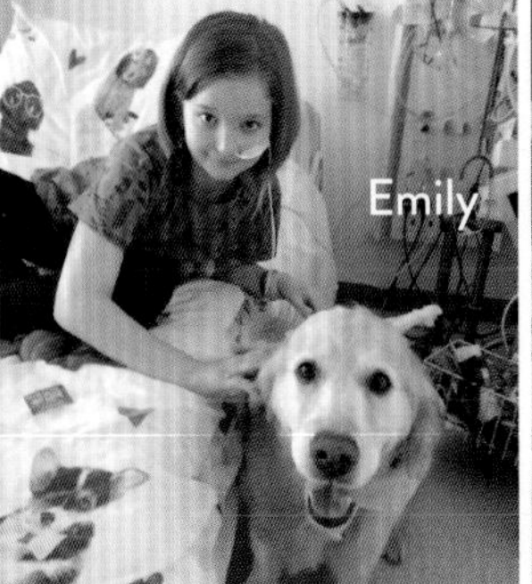
Emily

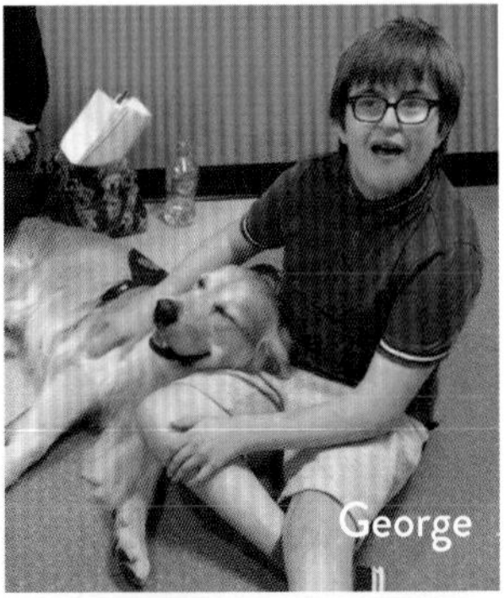
George

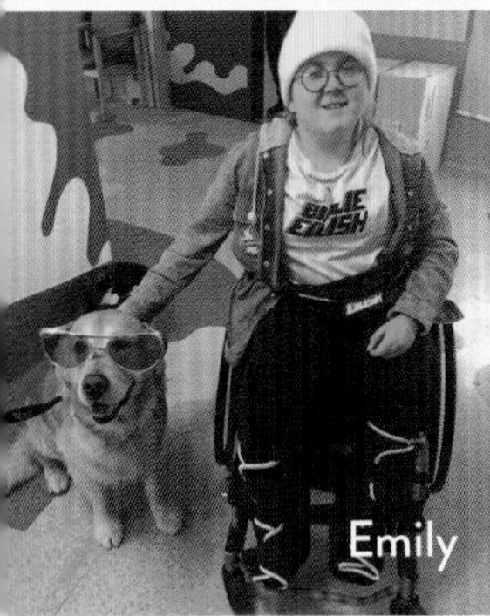
Emily

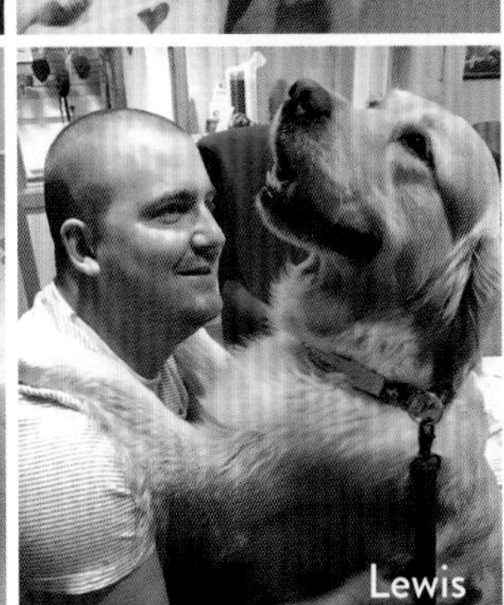
Lewis

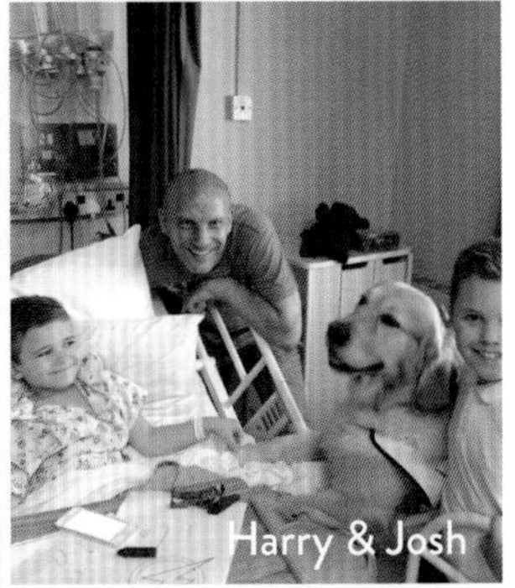
Harry & Josh

THESE ARE JUST SOME OF THE THOUSANDS OUR TEAM HAS SEEN!

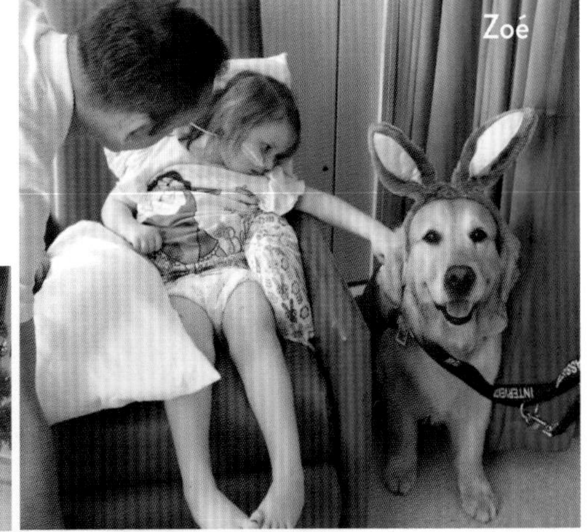
Zoé

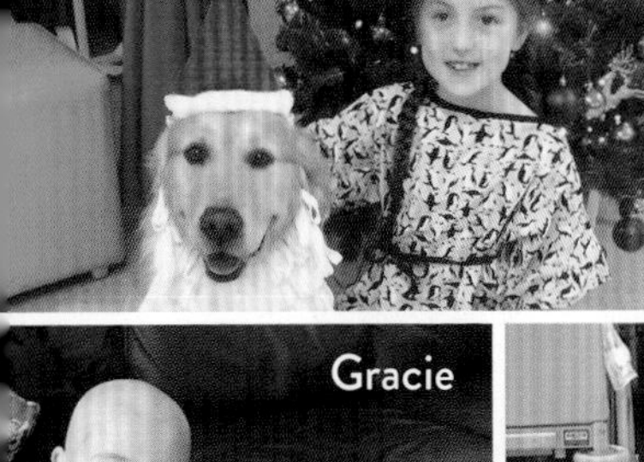
Annie

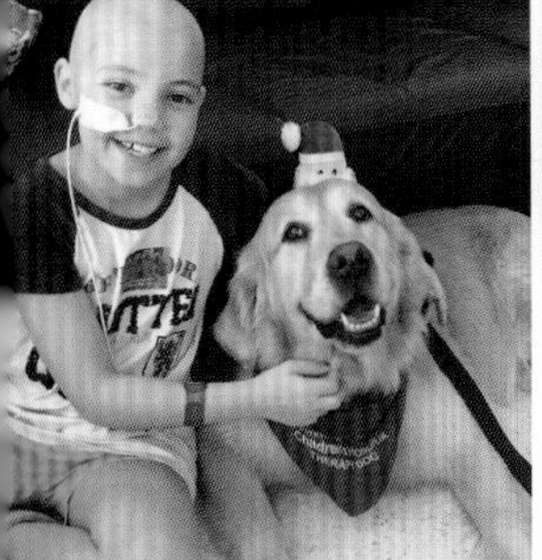
Gracie

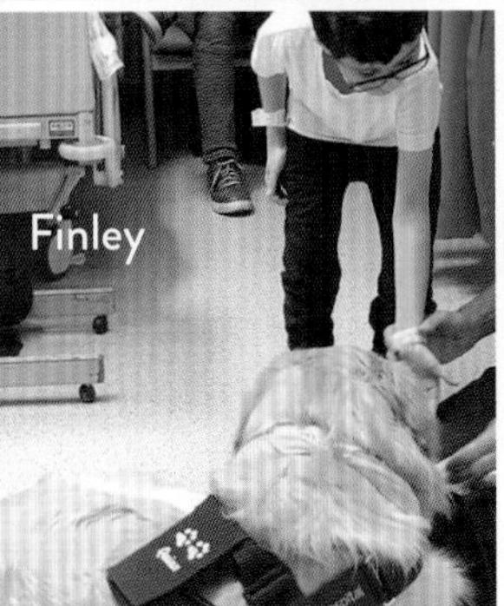
Finley

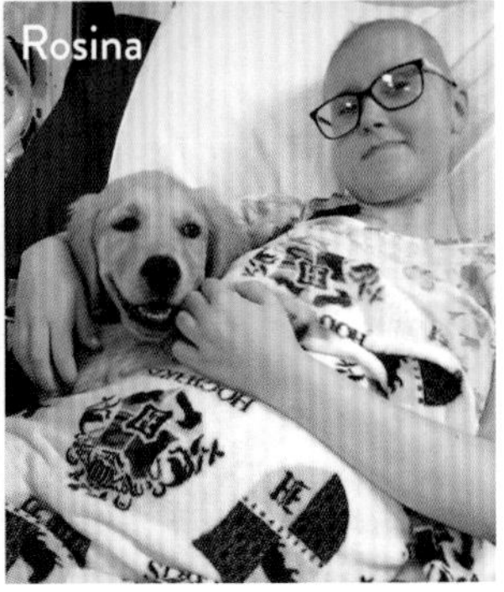
Rosina

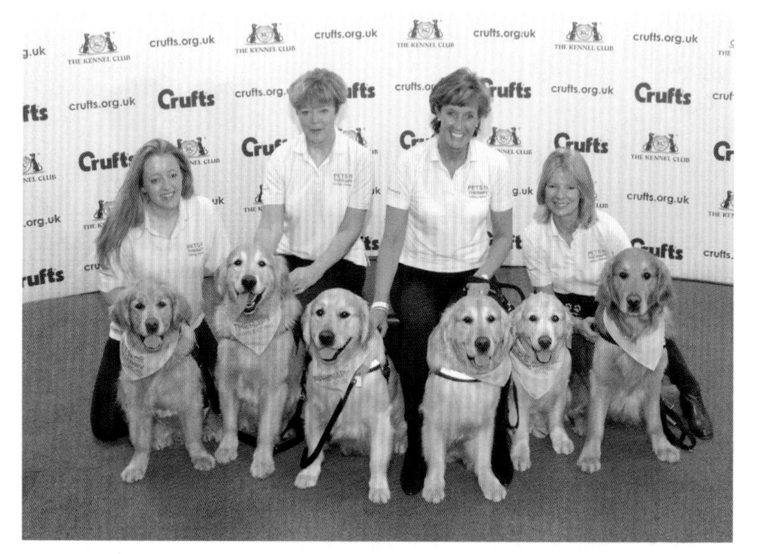

Our golden dream team at Crufts 2020.
From left to right – Humans: Hannah, Karen, me, Liz
Canines: Hattie, Archie, Quinn, Leo, Jessie, Milo.

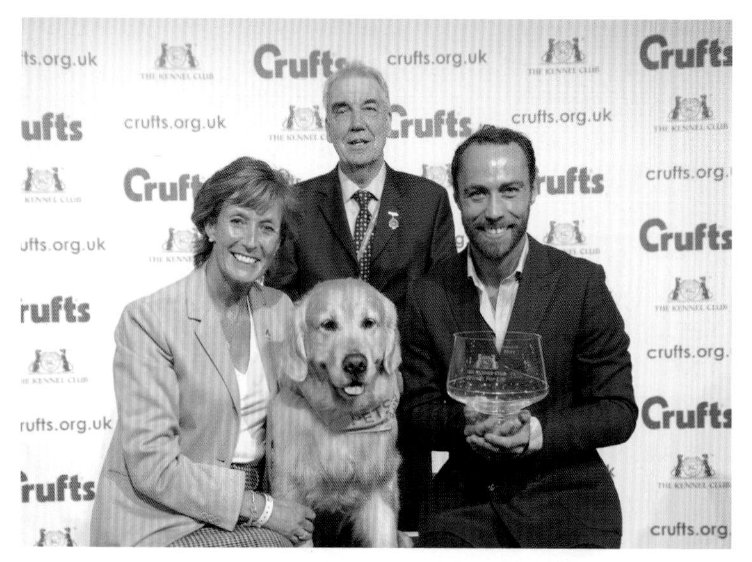

Me, Revd Bill King, the Chair of the KC Charitable Trust, and James Middleton. And Leo, of course!

back! The reply came right back: 'Yes, please!' And then, 'But I'd rather stroke you if I'm honest, love!' The ward was in uproar, staff and patients. I was still giggling to myself when I said: 'Thank you, sir, but only the dog is on offer today!'

Living and learning, I finished the visit, still laughing after the cheeky comment. You're lost without a sense of humour in the NHS and whatever role you have in a hospital, you have to be ready for the unexpected – especially if you have a dog by your side.

As I drove home that day, my mission to bring some canine joy to strangers on the wards of the hospital complete, I had a thought: Why had no one put in a request for a visit to a children's ward?

Thinking of how Ollie missed the dogs when he was in hospital, it was no great leap to imagine how many other children could perhaps enjoy seeing dogs. I decided that I needed to make that my next mission – to take the dogs to the children. And I knew that, in Leo, I had the perfect dog for such a special job.

Funny how they say: Be careful what you wish for. The very next time we checked in with Kim Sutton for our duties, we were asked to visit a patient on one of the general paediatric wards, whose parents had put in a request after seeing a therapy dog in the foyer. Another dog called Cognac had occasionally visited some of the children's wards but it would be great if we could do this request. I went up and saw the child and inevitably there were lots more who wanted to say hello too. A few weeks later I was invited onto the paediatric oncology ward. There it was, exactly what I wanted, a bigger way of giving back to that ward, but I was afraid. I wasn't sure if I could face it. I thought my days on that ward were well and truly over, apart from my occasional volunteering with their charity manager.

The first time Alice Razza reached for the warmth of a therapy dog's fur she was just 11 years old and the fur belonged to Monty. The first day that we were invited onto the paediatric oncology ward at SCH, I heard about Alice Razza or should I say, Alice heard about my therapy dogs, Monty and Leo, at the time. The sad thing was that she was simply too poorly to leave her room. I visited every week, sometimes with Monty and other times with Leo. We went to the playroom, where anyone who was well enough to see us was made most welcome and given a little slice of normal life outside the confines of the rooms on the hospital ward.

In those very early days of our hospital visits in 2013, we were not allowed into patients' rooms on the oncology ward, so there was no way I could get closer to Alice, even though I knew that seeing the dogs was likely to give her a massive lift. It was a very scary time for her and her parents, Debbie and Rik, who had been landed with the devastating diagnosis of their daughter's embryonal undifferentiated sarcoma, an extremely rare liver cancer. Every week we trotted in but there was no sign of Alice. We always passed a message through the nursing team to all the families that the dogs were around, but I wondered if a photograph of the nurses with Leo would help. Later, we heard Alice was overjoyed!

The day that Alice felt well enough to come and meet us was a big moment for everyone. It was a Monty day and that big old teddy of a dog sat patiently waiting for the touch of her outstretched hands. The smile on Alice's face lit up the room as she focused on Monty and reached out all of her fingers to eagerly sink into his golden coat. He looked so happy to have Alice looking him right in the eye, fussing him and loving him. Alice's mum took a picture and cried ... this time, she told me, with pure happiness. It had been a while since all the cancer business began that she had seen her daughter smile.

Alice did her very best to make it to our weekly visits. The dogs seemed to be a kind of medicine and nothing like the kind that came from a bottle. Monty and then Leo helped her face her illness by just being with her and helping her communicate more about her cancer and how to describe her feelings at all the different stages of her illness. The dogs did that. Alice had a stoic strength that so often defied belief.

The visits and the cuddles became the focus of smiles and when Alice relapsed in 2016, the cancer ripping into her ribs and lungs, she knew that her time was more precious than ever, so she made plans: '... I will make some great memories with everyone I love,' she told her family. And that list of loved ones included Leo and his friends who, by then, had become a fun and treasured part of her hospitalisation and ultimately her palliative care at home. Alice lived some of her short life in the shadow of cancer. It may have shortened her time on this earth, but she didn't allow it to take the joy out of her days.

So, how did it feel when I was asked to take my dogs into Piam Brown children's oncology ward? So many feelings raced towards me, all those weeks pacing corridors and running up and down the stairs worrying about Ollie made it a massive watershed moment.

But I had made a deal with myself and it had to be kept. I expected to feel dread as I started to spend more time there, but instead, I felt that I was going home.

13

Leo leads the way!

LITTLE ARCHIE ADAMS WAS UPSET AND DISTRESSED. The monitors showed it. Paralysed and confined to his hospital bed and only 18 months old – that was Archie's new world since being admitted a few days earlier. One of the matrons on the paediatric intensive care unit (PICU) saw me in the corridor and asked me if I could visit with Leo as she had seen how patients on some of the other wards had rallied just through the excitement of seeing the dogs walking around the ward. She wondered if Leo could work his magic for Archie in intensive care.

I had not met Archie before, or his parents who weren't there at the time, and when I found out that the family didn't have a dog at home, I really wasn't sure if we were going to be able to help a little boy who was so young. It seems odd to me now that I put so much emphasis on people already being familiar with dogs or being dog lovers as a yardstick for our chances of success with a patient. That was a big lesson learnt early on this journey – you don't have to share your home with a dog to love dogs, and once I realised that, I based my approach on three things:

trust, hope and the child not having any allergies or medical reason not to visit, in which case it had to be worth a try.

Archie was a tiny body with a head of golden curly hair lying in a big bed surrounded by heaps of hospital hardware. After contracting a virus, he had been left paralysed. While the medics worked out whether this was permanent or not, Archie was there amidst all the high-tech gadgetry testing to see what he could and couldn't do. There were so many teams trying to help him: doctors, nurses, physiotherapists ... too many to name. Pain, frustration, confusion and an element of isolation must have all been in the mix of feelings that Archie had running through him as he lay there with tubes and medication keeping him alive and unable to communicate. Only a few days earlier he had been toddling around a play park with his brother. Now he could only turn his head a tiny amount, giving him limited vision left and right, which meant that his only good view was of the ceiling tiles.

As we approached the bed Leo seemed to sense that his potential new patient needed him. He was not bothered by the huge bank of equipment or multiple people working to help Archie; that only made Leo more curious and I could tell by his eagerness to get closer that he wanted to close down the upset – I guess in the same way we humans feel the need to give someone a hug when they are sad. As we walked across with Matron, I hoped that we could bring Archie at least a little distraction and ultimately some comfort. I introduced myself to him, leaning in so that he could see me.

And then it was Leo's turn.

I hauled my 34kg fluffy partner into my arms to show Archie who had come to see him and asked if he would like Leo to come a bit closer. Archie's eyes widened, as if to say: 'Ooh, yes please.' I put Leo back down on all four paws and then, always the careful one, he let me position him close to the lowered bed and support him as he rested his paws on the protective cover. Leaning forward, I took Archie's little hand and placed it on my dog's big paw. From that moment I knew dogs could make a difference to children's lives. I knew it the moment I watched that little boy, exhausted by pain and sickness ... smile! I was seeing the connection between Archie and Leo for the first time. There it was, the spark created between a dog and a child. And in that moment I knew I was witnessing a little bit of canine magic!

I don't know what went on between Leo and Archie in those precious moments. All I know is that I was there supporting Leo at the bedside and very aware that I had witnessed something incredibly powerful. And I wasn't the only one to see it. The medical team watching the monitors recorded how the little one's vital signs improved. It was the first big indication to everyone involved in Archie's care that there was a way through to this little boy and perhaps that meant hope for better days ahead. And it all came about in the moment Archie and Leo looked into each other's eyes: it was like sunshine had shone into the room.

Later that day, Southampton Children's Hospital Twitter told of the good news: '*Amazing to hear today PICU nurses describe vital signs of boy in PICU calm and settled when Leo comes to visit @lyndseyuglow well done Leo xx*'.

Believe me, I couldn't wait to take Leo back to Archie's bedside. What happened wasn't imagined, it was real and it had my brain ticking over. I wondered if Leo could take this one step further – if he could help the clinical staff gauge the extent of Archie's paralysis. My mind started to run and over the next few months I found myself thinking more and more that there must be something we could do to help. At the same time the clinical teams tried all sorts of nerve condition studies and many other tests to see if they could generate a flicker of movement from those paralysed limbs. I wondered, maybe if I was permitted to put peanut butter on Archie's hands or feet and turned to Leo's expert licking skills, could we show if the nerves were active? It had to be worth a try if we could get special permission. After all, peanut butter will always get Leo's attention and if I encouraged him, he would surely do it despite knowing that he's not generally allowed to lick patients. But then they aren't normally covered in peanut butter!

I appreciate that my odd ideas can sometimes be seen as just that – a bit odd. But one day, after all other avenues had been exhausted, with the backing of Archie's parents and the paediatric physiotherapy team who were working with him, I happily spread a little peanut butter on our patient's right hand and then supported Leo at the bedside so he was able to lean in and do his stuff. I've no idea what Archie must have been thinking although I quietly explained every move as we went along and having learned to blink his acceptance and communicate with us all by now, he didn't seem at all phased by what happened next. Leo, being Leo, didn't waste any time getting 'licky and sticky'. There was a brief flicker between Archie's neck and shoulder on his right side. Now all we had to do was try to replicate it, but, sadly, it didn't come again that day.

It was an idea that did not require expensive technology ... just a jar of dog-friendly peanut butter and an inquisitive dog! It was not scientific but it had to be worth a try in a situation like Archie's. I would love to be able to say that there was a huge revelation, but all the neurological studies had shown the same: Archie had no activity in his limbs. He could see when he was touching the dog but sadly could not feel it. Another day, another try to see what could be done for their son; Archie's parents thanked me for trying the peanut butter anyway. I have discovered that's one of the stumbling blocks that parents of children with complex, hybrid serious illnesses are often faced with – a lengthy waiting period for diagnosis while the clinicians go to the ends of the earth to try to see what they can do for their patient. For Archie's parents the ultimate diagnosis was transverse myelitis and a permanent paralysis. It's a tough call, just waiting and waiting for answers, especially when you are helpless in the process and it's your child lying there. I know, I've been there myself, albeit not to the same extent, and I've seen it in other families, many times.

Having Leo beside me, I felt that I had a chance to bring something positive and Archie's case helped me to see that I was on the right track.

What had I started?

More importantly, where was this taking me?

My own experience had taught me that life in hospital is not an easy one; it's limiting for the child and for the siblings and parents too, which turns a distraction as tangible as a dog into something warm and responsive to literally hold onto. I was beginning to understand not just the comfort of canine company but its power too, especially when introduced to a very small child in an alien environment like a hospital. All my dogs visited Archie many times in the eighteen months he was on the wards. Every visit to a child teaches me something new and I do everything I can to adapt to help others. Archie taught me a huge amount. He was 18 months old, I was a stranger with a dog in an alien environment (PICU), where he was getting used to being cared for by a team he had only known a couple of days. The results on his intensive care monitors showed it worked; his vital signs improved.

He loved seeing the dogs and as time went on he would enjoy us visiting, but of course as he was unable to feel the dogs' fur, I had to try to create something different. When Archie was occasionally alone in the high dependency unit where he spent months, I would make up a toddler story and tell it to him with the dog as the hero. His eyes would light up and he would nod or blink enthusiastically at some of the fictional antics I described. There were occasions when the nurse looking after him would be writing up the documents at the end of the bed and I would realise she had heard some of the story and clearly thought I was quite mad, but it entertained a little chap when his parents couldn't always be there.

To me smiles are the best kind of medicine and the one reaction that dogs are almost guaranteed to gift on a visit. Leo taught me that a dog can adjust their energy in response to the child's condition. It's as if they sense the need to be ultra-calm in a very poorly child's presence. In Leo, it seems this is instinctive.

He always gives so much of himself. I've watched him and it is there with the children more than at any other time. He seems to know which patients need him most and those who are critically ill receive his special attention. He presents his paws to them on the pad on their bed, his head leaning in, offering a chance to touch, and then he brings a sense of calm, lowers his panting and stops moving his tail so that he doesn't rock the bed. At times, Leo can get so deep into his connection with a patient that he refuses to leave them. It's not unusual for me to be seen carrying him out of a ward or a child's room.

14

Giving back

NIXON HANSFORD LEFT HOSPITAL on Jersey at just one day old and was transferred to Southampton Children's Hospital. He was four months old when he met Leo for the first time in paediatric intensive care. The baby boy had just undergone a tracheotomy and had tubes protruding from all over his little body. He was scared, exhausted and had that faraway look children get when they have been in hospital a long time. And then ... in walked Leo. Now, I am just at one end of the lead doing the lifting and supporting, the star of the show is the dog. And Leo, again, knew exactly what to do: Nixon was in the arms of his mum, he looked at Leo and Leo offered the baby boy his head to stroke. There it was ... the connection.

Nixon didn't show any fear or anxiety even though he had never seen the outside world, let alone a dog before. His life thus far had been lived within the walls of the paediatric intensive care unit. And it was here that Leo became a regular visitor and comforter to both the little boy and his mum, when he was invited to wander into Nixon's bed space to spend some special time together enjoying a break from the normal hospital routine. I loved the fact that just taking the dog in to see her son I was able to give his mum someone to talk to for a few minutes too.

I held Leo in easy reach of Nixon as they enjoyed being close to each other. His mum and I looked at both of them as we chatted, convinced that boy and dog had their own language in their silence. Leo always moved his head closer to Nixon to make it easy for his friend to give him attention, which worked really well and encouraged movement. In turn, in his eagerness to make the most of each visit, as Nixon became stronger, he went on to make a big effort to sit up so that he could interact with Leo.

With each visit, there was progress and smiles, there are always smiles when Leo is around. Every time that happens in the presence of parents it is super-special, especially when it happens during a long period of treatment, because we can all work together to do what we can to help support them as well as their child through the worst of times. Under the guidance and the blessing of the clinical staff, we all have a place on the team. For me, it's sharing Leo so that everyone witnesses the benefit of having a dog on the wards. And this is exactly what happened with Nixon; it was such a privilege to be a part of his care.

It was seven months before Nixon was well enough to go home to Jersey, but his ongoing treatment meant that our paths would cross several times more and we got to meet his brother and dad too. Leo, it seems, had become quite a talking point in the Hansford family. In our many times together at her son's bedside, Nixon's mum said that the whole experience with Leo made her son less anxious in what was a very worrying situation for the whole family. Meeting Leo, she told me, was: 'a tear-jerking moment and an amazing one', and those moments were repeated many more times as Nixon grew and learnt to live with his genetic condition. It is wonderful to see him growing up – and now the family have their own dog too. When we spoke about me writing this book, his mum told me with pride that Nixon chose to 'sign' Leo's name before anyone else's and at seven years old is still talking about Leo. Leo, the people-pleaser, was starting to gain his own fan club!

In those early days on the wards, I realised that for some people a big part of what we were doing had little more than a novelty value. After all, the perceived 'therapy' was given by big, friendly, shaggy-coated, gold-coloured dogs, so it was inevitable that they were going to attract attention no matter what we were up to. That's why I had to make sure that we were seen to be up to something good, something worthwhile.

Once in the building, people would do double-takes watching the dog trotting along to the wards and some of the onlookers were parents wondering if their child could benefit from a visit from a dog. Although whichever one was with me – Monty, Leo, Jessie or Totty – was always in their PAT working jacket, they were still a dog taking a stroll and it is pretty rare to have something as 'normal' as that in a hospital. Just catching sight of the dog was enough to break up what can potentially be very dull, worrisome days with little or no distraction from the focus of illness.

It became clear that in most cases, a visit from a dog could bring comfort to a child, or for that matter, to an adult, so maybe, in hindsight, it is no surprise that requests for visits began to pile in from all directions. Most reassuring for me was that we were starting to receive requests not only from interested parents but from the clinical teams too.

I started to feel that things were about to get busier. I had all four dogs on the rota: on Tuesdays we visited the hospital and then on Thursdays we would visit the care homes, alternating them so we went fortnightly; I had it all covered. I loved visiting the hospital so much that if I could fit in an extra visit I would, but it wasn't always possible. In the hospital, at this time, we were anywhere and everywhere across the adult wards based on the requests the volunteers' office had received. After our initial visits to Alice and others, we were making an in-road with the children's wards too. But being so busy was fine because I like things to be that way and I didn't want to let anything go or let anyone down when my dogs were just beginning to make an impression.

One of the biggest jobs I had from day one was keeping on top of the dogs' cleaning and clipping regime. Every visit was to a clinical environment and to make a success of this mission of mine, the onus was on me to maintain a robust doggy wash-and-go routine. I have always been aware that it is a privilege to be allowed onto the wards and, even when you know you are doing something good and helping others, it's wise to accept that potential critics lurk in most corners. Leo and his friends are big, hairy dogs, that's true, but when the infection control team know that they have enjoyed a warm dog shower and the blaster dryer at home, followed by sitting in their doggy dressing gowns, they agree that my salon lovelies are consistently clean enough to walk the wards. I am sure my neighbours must sometimes wonder what I am doing on the other side of the fence! But then, as most dog owners know, living with dogs has its crazy moments.

What do they say about working with children and animals? I love Leo and there is nothing he could ever do to make me think differently. I just sometimes wish he didn't have such a stubborn streak! For a dog who has never been driven by food, it turns out that he is a four-legged pain in the bottom to drag past a hospital cake sale. It started one day with a small flapjack offered by a kind volunteer from her trestle table full of goodies in the hospital foyer. Of course, I blame myself for what happened next. As soon as that flapjack was guzzled by Leo, he added a new handy fact to his brain file: 'Trestle table means treat'! To this day, Leo remains distracted by a trestle table. No matter why it happens to be in the hospital foyer and whether or not it is an information stand or there is food, he still insists on sitting patiently beside it in the vain hope that he will receive a treat. Until then, we can't pass!

My otherwise well-behaved golden retriever is never short of attention from the moment we arrive at the hospital. I must admit to feeling enormously proud of him and of all my brood. I have rarely had to apologise for their behaviour and when I do, it's never their fault. This reminds me of a saying my dad had: 'You can take them anywhere twice, and the second time is to apologise.' He first used that when Harry and Ollie were toddlers but he decided it applied to our dogs too! For instance, the only reason they all stop to check out the entrance to M&S on the way out of the hospital is because a grateful parent once decided to treat them to a box of cocktail sausages right outside the store – they have never forgotten it!

My pact with myself was, I thought, going well. I was paying back and everyone was loving the dogs, but I still had a nagging doubt that I wasn't doing enough. My dogs were more than doing their bit, in every little flash of their special personalities they were helping patients make memories. I only had one concern and that was for Totty. She loved the care home visits because she loved elderly people, but she didn't have Monty's patience or Leo's sensitivity in the hospital's intensive care environment. Totty was more of a speed-dater, like Jessie, and perfect for the meeting, greeting and moving on style of visit, but sitting by someone's bedside for a longer period to talk or help with an aspect of their care was never really her style. It took me a couple of years to work out why Totty was at her happiest with care home residents before the penny dropped – it was the lack of syringe pumps.

In care homes she didn't have to work around any medical equipment to do her thing and the residents loved her instantly. The stage was hers without any complications or competition and her audience was sat ready and waiting for her moment to mingle, mooch and generally entertain! She did continue to visit some of the general wards at the hospital and the playrooms if I needed her, but she never went back to oncology, high dependency, or intensive care once I had worked out where she was at her happiest.

In a way, I was relieved that Totty had made her preference known and I was OK with it because I had Leo, Jessie and Monty for the hospital element of our rota and that was all working perfectly. At least, that's what I thought until the day in 2013 when Leo fell ill.

I came downstairs to let the dogs out and was horrified to see that Leo couldn't walk and he was obviously in a good deal of pain. I contacted our vet, Alex, immediately and after a home visit she knew he needed an X-ray so we lifted him into the car. She quickly got the tests underway to help find out what was wrong. I didn't want to believe this was happening. Blood tests and X-rays didn't throw up anything conclusive, no bones were showing signs of injury. Alex said to keep him comfortable and that she would review him the next morning.

He was in so much pain he had to be supported if he wanted a pee. The rest of his time was spent sitting with me trying to tempt him to eat something but he'd never had the best of appetites. I was doing my best to keep us both comfortable when Mike came home. I was in pieces. I tried to explain what was going on and what had been said but Mike was already examining Leo – checking every limb as if the dog was one of his young patients. He had a suspicion that it was something he had seen previously in children, but of course they were usually able to say where it hurt. With Leo it was not so easy, but Mike did get a response when he exerted a little pressure between two of the dog's vertebrae. He called Alex to share his thoughts and both decided that the symptoms were a fit for a bacterial infection involving one of the intervertebral discs (discs in his spine), a condition called discospondylitis, which is known as discitis in humans. They decided that Leo must go on antibiotics right away.

It was horrible seeing Leo so poorly and when told that it could take four to six weeks for him to fully recover, I felt so guilty. I knew that it wasn't my fault because nothing anyone had done made this happen and he was certainly receiving the best of veterinary care, but it was the first big red flag for me – seeing how other people reacted to Leo not being on the wards. Other people were growing to love him and rely on him at the hospital. I knew that I had to get him through this for all of us who couldn't bear to watch him suffer, but mostly I had to do this for *my* Leo.

Recovery was a long, slow process. And at first, he seemed fine with all the lying around and being cuddled, but after a few weeks even our lazy boy Leo wanted to get up and out and no doubt back to his visiting duties. Patience is certainly not one of my virtues, but I had no choice this time. Every day as I watched Leo improve, I thought how good it would be to have him padding through the corridors of the hospital again. I was still visiting with my other dogs but I knew that some of the staff and some of his regular patients were asking when he would be back. They were missing him.

When Leo was finally able to be back on duty, it was such a relief. He was usually fairly reluctant to get in the back of the car, something that probably harks back to his first experience as our puppy passenger from France, but after his enforced break he gained a little spring in his step as if he was eager to be on the thirteen-mile journey to the hospital once again.

15

Meeting Jo and Dylan: a new direction

STAFF REQUESTS FOR OUR VISITS TO CHILDREN were building and that's exactly what I hoped would happen. To see the smiles that the dogs were bringing to patients, parents and staff was just incredible. Again, I really felt that my paying back was genuinely happening. Demand was still coming from all over the hospital, but I was achieving my wish to spend more time with the children and so our days were mostly spent moving around the children's hospital wards. The day we met Jo Faulks our work with therapy dogs went in a new and unexpected direction.

Leo and I first met Jo at the Macmillan Centre as dogs were not allowed in the Teenage and Young Adults cancer ward, something that sadly has not changed. Kim Sutton, the voluntary services manager, had asked me to see her following a request from her parents. All I knew about Jo that day was that she was 24, a dog lover and that she was receiving care for a cancer which was now in its advanced stages.

Fed up with her wispy hair and people staring, Jo decided to shave her head and create a bucket list that included holding a puppy – and a golden retriever was her favourite breed. I guessed that is where we came in, although at the time we did not have puppies so Leo had to step in as the big, soft, cuddly flump that he is. It was a lovely visit. Leo was perfectly gentle and attentive to his new friend, which meant she was able to enjoy his calm company without tiring too quickly. They were happy together and Jo was smiling so when her dad thanked me for the visit and for raising Jo's spirits, it was my pleasure to agree to visit again the following week. It was in making the arrangements for that second visit that her dad revealed that Jo was suffering from the same type of leukaemia that Ollie had survived. The words acute myeloid leukaemia hit me in the stomach like a fist.

I made the arrangements but ended up thinking about it again a few hours later as I wondered whether this was something I could really do. It suddenly felt too close, too personal. Was it going to be too painful a reminder? Jo was experiencing a relapse – something I had dreaded from the moment my son was given the all-clear and here I was again staring AML in the face. I had already agreed but now I was questioning what on earth I was doing. Was this too close for comfort? Come on, Lyndsey, I said to myself, it was time to dig deep and besides, how would I feel if someone had let Ollie down? I had to do it; after all, wasn't he the reason that I was doing this work with the therapy dogs in the first place? To help others, to bring them comfort where I could?

The arranged visit triggered a few sleepless nights when my fears of Ollie relapsing ran away with themselves. All I could see was a family suffering just as we had suffered, but there was a big difference – Ollie was home and well. I told myself: I can do this. I went to see Jo again in the Macmillan Centre with Leo and it was another wonderful visit, where the obvious connection between Leo and Jo brought her such peace and laughter. As we left, I promised we would make it happen again.

Jo was so poorly but she always found enough energy from somewhere to enjoy a little cuddle-time with Leo. I wanted her to enjoy every second with the dogs and that was totally possible while she was in hospital but things became more of a challenge when she left to continue her palliative care at home. I was forced to rethink how I was going to keep my promise to Jo. I had to find a way because Jessie was due to have puppies in July and I wanted Jo to be able to hold a pup, just as she had wished for on her bucket list. The problem was now she was at home, a visit there was not covered by PAT insurance.

Undeterred, I started calling insurers. I didn't stop until I found one able to accept me for private public liability cover for working dogs and took out the policy immediately. It was only right, I felt that I needed to do this for Jo and I felt it even more earnestly when I took Leo to see her at her home.

It was there I told her that Jessie was expecting pups and that in a few weeks she would hopefully be able to see them, but that we must introduce her to Jessie before that time to help them build a relationship before she whelped her litter.

Popping round to Jo's house and spending time with her and her family was an incredible experience. She was a very brave young woman who taught me so much about facing your fears. She had a way about her that was so wise and knowing and the closer we became to the family, the more we all hoped that Jo would be with us to see Leo and Jessie's pups into the world.

Of course, the world doesn't present just one hurdle at a time and 2014 was proving to be no different. The day after Jessie's scan confirmed she was pregnant, Harry called me to say that he was in with a chance of being selected for the GB Junior Rowing Team and that training was going really well but it would be several weeks before he would know if he would be on the final team list. Meanwhile, I kept in touch with Jo and invited her to our home to see all of the dogs: we even managed to arrange a surprise visit from a friend's golden retriever pup, Barney, who at 12 weeks old was full of mischief and gave Jo so many reasons for laughing out loud.

There was so much going on at home and with the visits to our patients in hospital and Jo at home, I was afraid everything was going to happen all at the same time, leaving me with some big decisions to make. And I was right. Harry, aged 17, was selected to row for the GB Junior Rowing Team at the Coupe de la Jeunesse in France and Jessie had her litter of ten pups on 22 July!

As soon as the first pup arrived, I messaged Jo's parents to say they were on the way and that I would keep them posted. They replied that Jo was at the hospital having a blood transfusion. It was all happening! As the deliveries started to slow towards the end of the whelping, I sent a message to say that I felt sure she had one more but the others had arrived and sent a picture. I told them that if they wanted to pop round on the way home, they were welcome, and besides, Jo and Jessie had become good friends over the weeks of visiting. As luck would have it, Jo arrived just as the last pup was born. It was magical to see her smile. Once we had made sure Jessie and all the puppies were safe and well, I passed one of the earliest born to Jo and there she was with a pup in her hands, another tick on her bucket list completed.

Jo and her parents were given an open invitation to pop round and see the pups whenever suited them. After all, I wasn't going anywhere … I would be with the pups 24/7 to watch over them and make sure Jessie had everything she needed. Jo was unwell but determined to keep up her visits to our home every few days to see the pups. Sometimes she was so weak that she was close to being carried through our front door, but once in, she was happy lying in a reclining chair with a pup on her chest as she drifted in and out of sleep. On better days she had enough energy to enjoy the pups' antics minute by minute. I know now that we were all witnessing Animal Assisted Intervention at its purest. Jo was so happy and hundreds of pictures were taken by her boyfriend and parents to capture those precious memories.

Seven days later I took a call from Jo's dad, asking if she could come visit the pups as it was her birthday and it was the one thing that she definitely wanted to do. I said yes and quickly sent one of the boys out to get some flowers so that when Jo arrived, Jessie, who loves to carry a gift for guests, could take them to the front door to greet her. Jo had little energy that day but she was happy lying with Boris, one of the sleepier pups, on her chest while she drifted between sleep and waking. In between her snoozes we chatted and Jo smiled as she gently caressed the pup, while around her the other pups were enjoying cuddles from her parents and her boyfriend, who all appeared in need of the warm, furry distraction. As the family left, I had to tell them that I would be heading out on the last flight on Friday to watch Harry compete in France that weekend but not to worry as the pups would be in the care of our vet Alex, who had taken time off and was moving into the house while we were away. I wanted them to know that all they had to do was call to say that they were bringing Jo over and it would be OK. I said all that, but somehow, I knew they wouldn't and in my heart I wondered, as I closed the door, if I had seen Jo for the last time.

I felt awful. I didn't want my trip, creating memories with my own family, to prevent Jo and her family having more last puppy cuddles. I told myself that I had done all I could to make sure Jo could see the pups whenever she wanted, knowing that Alex would make everyone welcome if she came, but of course ... she didn't. That weekend Jo sadly passed away.

It happened while I was celebrating Harry's silver medal in the single sculls for Great Britain. I was home by the time Jo's parents gave me the news and asked me whether I would be around over the next few weeks when the funeral was due to take place. I felt so dreadful when I had to say that I was already booked to go to Florida to volunteer at Give Kids the World with Ollie. I understand that her service was a beautiful celebration of everything Jo loved about life and a few weeks later her parents came round for coffee and told me that the celebration included a video of many aspects of Jo's life ... including Leo and Jessie's pups.

Leo loved his time with Jo at the hospital and for me it was an absolute honour and pleasure to be able to transfer her time with the dogs from hospital to home. It was our first home palliative care case and I was aware that this had not been done by any of the therapy dogs at Southampton before. This was a ground-breaking move, one that didn't go unnoticed. To me it was just a case of doing the right thing for the patient. We did it to keep a promise to a young woman whose last wish was to hold a golden retriever puppy before she died. I didn't think that was a lot to ask, I still don't.

But that's what happens when dogs and families come together and there is trust and a commitment to palliative care.

I remember Dylan Vanhear as a brave young man who loved Leo very much. From the moment they met, 11-year-old Dylan saw my dog not just as his friend but also his fellow conspirator! The relationship between the two of them always caused a few laughs as a therapy dog was one of the only things that could be guaranteed to encourage Dylan to take a break from his love of video games.

Dylan was trapped by the painful effects of a spinal tumour and all the frustrations associated with life at the children's hospital, stuck there for a total of 308 days. The special adaptations to his home were taking longer than expected, so even as his active treatment came to an end his parents were unable to make plans to take him out of what Dylan saw as his prison. If there was one place this boy didn't want to be it was in hospital, confined to his room. It was no wonder then that one day when we arrived on the ward, he was getting very stressed because the staff wanted to take his electric wheelchair for servicing. Dylan was making it very clear that he really didn't want that to happen. Being without the independence of that wheelchair was his worst nightmare and, I think, he was afraid that if they took it, they would not bring it back.

In total panic, Dylan attempted a quick getaway only to be stopped in his tracks by a flat battery and a wall of people trying to persuade him back to his room. Angry, out of pure frustration, he let rip with a tirade of expletives aimed at anyone who was listening. I was walking towards him and his poor parents looked so embarrassed but it was water off a duck's back to me. Never one to shy away, I leant over and whispered in Dylan's ear: 'You can't effing swear on the ward but you can swear at Leo if you whisper very quietly.' Dylan burst out laughing and, in an instant, that was him back to the old Dylan, all cuddles and squeezes being given to Leo. We went back to his room with him, the wheelchair went off for service and all was well.

I truly believe there was something in Leo's calm way that connected with the boy's pain and frustration throughout his long time at the hospital. Leo simply didn't change or react to the noise or the behaviour, he just stuck to being

Leo pushing aside the anger and seeing through the fear to the boy. And that's the place where, I believe, they met right back at the beginning of his treatment in the neurological ward – boy meets dog and they go on to have fun together. It's so simple in one way, but otherworldly in another. The laughter and the calmness that just happened whenever the two met was, I admit, heart-breaking, particularly as his prognosis became evident. I can't explain it, but I know that something good happened in Leo's journey with Dylan. Over time, he met all of the therapy dogs but still had his favourite.

It had been Dylan's consultant who ventured the idea that an intervention by Leo could ease the boy's pain when he was in hospital and then we were able to transfer over to the hospice too when he went there for some respite care. Dylan missed Leo between visits as any one of us misses something that makes us smile. What he needed to ease his pain and frustration the dogs keyed into. That's how it worked and why Leo was such a big part of that healing partnership – they were lads together. They appeared together on *BBC South Today*, with Dylan giving away Leo's 'secrets'! And when Dylan spent a day with us at *Crufts* in 2016 (where Leo was a finalist for another award), he had to stay in hospice accommodation near the National Exhibition Centre the night before so that his care requirements could be fulfilled before he could come and support us in the finals, but it was a day he definitely was not going to miss. In amongst all the excitement of the event where he saw Leo first in the showring, then as a finalist in the PAT Dog of the Year competition, and ultimately met the Supervet, Noel Fitzpatrick, Leo was beside Dylan, helping him make memories that had nothing to do with cancer.

Leo and I attended Dylan's funeral. Even then, my amazing dog was his giving self as he led the mourners in with Dylan's brother Callum and later broke the ice between people, some of whom were children attending their first funeral. As Dylan's mother said: 'Leo seemed to understand the occasion and comforted the people who needed him most.'

Leo's special qualities as a therapy dog were clear for all the medical staff to see and not just within the confines of a visit, but in the never-ending relationships that developed between the dog and the families. He has a way with him that I was really only just fully appreciating. It was more than the special way he has of standing on his back legs with his front paws going instinctively towards the protective pad on the bed, which is a very handy addition to his great bedside manner. It was also being there to help in palliative care, another place where a therapy dog like Leo can make a world of difference in those precious last days and hours. Like all other aspects of what we do, it's about making memories. Watching a child near the end of their days and their parents' helplessness as the time slips away is hard and haunting every time. For me, sharing my therapy dogs and seeing them bring a blend of joy, distraction and a sense of normality onto a ward, to nourish the afraid and vulnerable, is an incredible feeling. It feels as if this is my purpose, my reason for being and it is certainly part of my reason for having multiple dogs.

There is something very special about the bond between the dogs and the young patients – the dogs being an important 'bridge' to the treatment process. And I realised that I was not the only one aware of what was happening: now the clinical teams were seeing it too. Leo was making an impression and was in even greater demand and I found it almost impossible to refuse any request for his presence – and Leo was more than happy with that.

I kept my promise to the Coopers and to myself to return to Give Kids the World in Florida as a volunteer with Ollie. We had a great time catching up with many of our old volunteer friends and colleagues as well as meeting new families with 'Wish' children. It's an incredibly special place that connects you with many of the emotions that many parents have to push into a place inside just to be able to function day to day. While there, it was no surprise to me that my thoughts turned to Jo Faulks and her family.

On the day of Jo's funeral, between volunteer shifts, I took myself to the non-denominational chapel where people can share their memories in books. I wanted to write Jo's name and the words 'thinking of you' but I didn't feel I could as these books were for families and their own 'Wish' children. I couldn't help feeling guilty for not being with the Faulks family that day, so the calm of the chapel was good and I spent a few minutes reading entries. In the thirty minutes before Ollie and I started our next shift, we walked to the 'Castle of Miracles' together and silently looked up at Ollie's star on the ceiling ... it had been there since we visited as a family, with him as a 'Wish' child, in

2009. As the tears flowed, I hugged him and knew that I was a lucky mum to have my boy with me and I felt thankful that I could give Jo her final wish to hold a puppy.

When I called Mike and Harry later that day to check in on the pups, I was still emotional about our time looking at Ollie's star and shared how, in that moment, my thoughts had turned to Jo. We ended our call counting our blessings.

16

Dogs working miracles!

'PLEASE DON'T EVER CHANGE, LYNDSEY, what you're doing with Leo, you're making such a difference!' When the UHS volunteer manager of the time, Kim Sutton, offered me those amazing words of encouragement I don't think she could have had any idea how much I needed to hear them or how well timed they were. Despite the fact that all my dogs were visitors, Kim recognised that he was extra special. She had nominated Leo for PAT Dog of the Year during the autumn of 2015 and the media waggon rolled swiftly into town.

If there was anyone in the hospital who had not met or heard about Leo the therapy dog, they were soon going to, thanks to the local TV and radio coverage which made him something of a four-pawed celebrity. Having such a great dog in my company, I was well used to people approaching and wanting to give him a hug, and full of questions about his name and, noticing his work jacket, asking: 'So, what does your PAT dog do, exactly?'

In some ways the media coverage saved me explaining over and over the role of the charity, the dogs and how Leo came to be nominated for the award, but to be honest I didn't mind at all. I was so proud of Leo and it was Kim recognising his special work, especially with very poorly children, that resulted in the nomination. Of course, all the attention triggered more requests from staff who were witnessing the breaking down of old apprehensions and barriers concerning the safety and benefit of dogs on hospital wards. The big positives were starting to melt away the old negatives because the great results were right in front of them.

Leo was smashing it! And we were busier than ever at the hospital.

I was striding, Leo pace – so not very fast at all – past the adult intensive care unit when I met a woman who told me that she was about to go onto the ward to see her husband. I stopped and we talked briefly. Sophie Aitkens told me that her husband was in an induced coma and intubated with a tube. I put an arm round her as I imagined the horror of seeing someone you love so vulnerable and offered to go in with her as a support if she thought it would help. Leo looked eager to go through the door. He was familiar with what went on with patients behind it and Sophie leant forward and stroked him for a bit of comfort before we went in. Once we had the consent of the team looking after him, I positioned Leo as close as I could to Barry, Sophie's husband, as he lay there and although I did not expect any response, it was amazing to see his hand move slowly when we put it on Leo's paw.

Sophie said: 'It was like seeing a snippet of Barry, not just a patient linked to a machine in a hospital bed. And, having two young children at home who were unable to visit their dad in hospital, it was so comforting to be able to tell them about Leo's visit and that made them smile and cry happy tears to know Leo made their dad's hand move. Leo took the scary out of a scary situation and I don't think anyone else could have done that for us at that horrible time.'

A few months later I was so surprised to run into Sophie again on the same hospital corridor. I recognised her straight away and, I'll admit, that my heart sank for a second, wondering what had brought her back to the hospital. Barry had been re-admitted and once again was in an induced coma. She asked me if I could take Leo in again as having him there before was such a wonderful thing and of course I agreed on the spot. Our visit could not have been timed more perfectly – we stepped into the room just a few minutes after Barry had been woken from the coma; his breathing tube had just been taken out, he was still on oxygen, but as soon as he saw Leo, he pulled off his mask and moved his face towards the dog ... and he cried.

It was quite a moment to witness. To be there with a family going through hell on earth and being able to bring some comfort through Leo was an absolute privilege. A long time later, talking to his family, Barry said that he had memories of a dog being with him during his first coma and felt calm and comforted as if he was home with their own dog. Sophie wrote to say how Leo gave that comfort to Barry in hospital and how that relationship had comforted them all in different ways: how he was the perfect distraction for their children, who came to see Leo as their dad's guardian while they couldn't visit him, and his presence connected the adults too. Leo was a vehicle for communication while they were apart and at Barry's bedside. I'm not sure how it works, but I know that it does. I was convinced that I had seen therapy dog magic in action with the Aitkens family, and I still believe it now.

The phrase 'making a difference' is banded about regularly these days and in connection with many things and it's not always apparent what 'difference' has been achieved or even if it counts for anything in the way it was promised. That's where I have the advantage, because, thanks to my dogs, I see that difference every time we visit patients. And the difference the dogs make rarely centres on just the patient in the bed, it's so very much about family. But fate is the master of the curved ball and when Mike asked me to step in on one of his young patients, I found myself counting my blessings a million times over … and then a million more as I held Leo closer.

It was an horrific car crash that left Jake, at eight years old, an orphan with catastrophic life-changing injuries. Mike operated on the extensive skeletal damage, but his concerns for this patient went beyond the physical as he knew this lad would have so much to deal with once he knew the extent of what had happened. The boy's mood remained low after the surgery while he recovered in the paediatric intensive care unit. Mike wondered if a visit from Leo just might be the best medicine to cheer up a very depressed boy. I was only ever going to say yes to his request. That's not because it was Mike who had asked me to help – I would have done the same for any team with a child in that situation – but because I knew that he could be right. Leo might just be the answer, or at least his presence could trigger a response of some kind. Anything to engage with Jake's emotions, which shock had most likely locked down. As ever, it was worth a try.

It was almost impossible for our patient to move, so I took Leo as near as I could to his bedside, the pad already in place for my dog's paws to rest on. We were all set, but I could never have imagined the moment that young boy, in all his misery and pain, reached out to touch Leo, moving his fingers slowly over his paw as if he were reaching for fingers to hold. Leo, perfectly still and, as ever, enjoying the attention of the clinical team looking on, was showcasing all that was good about the human-animal bond in that moment. At the same time the glimmer of a smile came into the boy's eyes. His face may have been swollen and contorted with injury, but through that his eyes smiled.

That's another beautiful thing about dogs: no matter what your circumstances, or injuries, your personal insecurities ... they never look shocked and they certainly never judge. Jake's swollen face and broken body did not stop Leo showing the boy affection. Leo was the same as he always is – a dog. A dog who somehow knows what to do.

In Jake's case, I wondered if Mike and I saw one of our own sons lying there helpless and remembered how Ollie felt trapped in hospital and cut off from the dogs' company. We'd both recognised the positive psychological turnaround in our son after he had seen Monty and Totty in the visit to the car park. If it worked for our child, surely a dog's intervention could work for someone else's? It was worth a try.

Once I realised that I had dogs who were so well suited to visiting children, I had a reason to continue to forge a path to work on the paediatric wards. Had they not been suited to the work, it would not have been ethical for me to do so. After all, I am only one half of the team, the dog makes the partnership. I always say, 'Handler desire may not always equate to canine ability': I can only do this if my dogs are suited to it and enjoy it.

I was then, and I am now, driven to do what I do. It comes from somewhere inside me. Is it personal passion that drives me? Or the power of: 'There but for the grace of God'? I don't know. Does it matter? All I know is that I have to do this and for as long as I have a dog that enjoys it, I will.

Whenever we visited Jake in the time that he was in hospital, Leo was just so gentle, exactly what he needed to be to bring calm and comfort. I admit there was something hugely rewarding in the fact that Mike had requested that Leo and I visit another one of his cases. This from a consultant orthopaedic surgeon, never mind being my husband and one of those who was initially wary of dogs visiting patients. In my mind it was a mark of approval – that he really believed that what I was doing had therapeutic benefits to patients. He had seen it with his own eyes with a number of patients by now but Jake was different. He had bad news coming about the loss of his parents and to be able to offer him Leo to hug was very moving for me.

Support from my family is massively important to me. I always needed their approval on all levels because everything I did affected all of us and, perhaps more importantly, it was on Mike's own hospital turf. I understood his early reticence. After all, the dogs are part of our family and he was massively aware of how they loved to chase squirrels, roll in muck and do all those unpredictable and often smelly things. That's why, when one of them did something typically 'doggy' in the hospital, I cringed big-time.

When I was given permission to take a future medical student on one of my hospital visiting rounds, I wondered if there was an ulterior motive. First of all, it wasn't something we normally did, but then her father was one of the doctors at the hospital and he was aware of the benefit we had on the patients. I took Leo as he was the star of the team and, overall, my most reliable dog, plus we had a lot of patients that he had been visiting on the wards at the time.

Once her lengthy student sign-in process was completed we headed straight for the wards as I was eager to show off what we did best. Buoyed partly by the student's interest and, as usual, by the attention from the patients, we spent longer there than usual doing our thing. This was ahead of my formal AAI training and learning the many, and necessary, ways of saying 'No'!

Visits concluded, we left the children's wards at the top of the hospital and took the lifts back to the ground floor, where Leo showed signs that he was ready to head out the door and head for home. And his needs are always my priority.

As we passed the cashpoint, a mother recognised us, leant out of the queue and asked if her son could say hello to Leo. Not wanting to disappoint her little one, who was there in his wheelchair, I said yes and she asked if they could have a photo as she hadn't taken one when they'd met before. Straight away I went into my routine when posing Leo for photos – he is very obliging – but as he was about to take up his sitting position ... out popped a small poo! OMG, the horror! We were in a busy corridor, so I super-quickly whipped out a poo bag, Meg (the student) rushed to the anti-bacterial hand gel dispenser and to get some paper towels. Within less than 120 seconds it was fully cleared up, but it felt like a lifetime. All three of us made a sharp exit and I took Leo to his usual place of relief to finish off, vowing never again! My father's saying was running through my head yet again: 'You can take the dogs anywhere twice and the second time is to apologise' and that was followed by Catherine's saying: 'It is never the dog, always the owner.'

Needless to say, I didn't sleep a wink that night. All I could think about was who I should report it to. I spoke to a senior member of the hospital team the next time I was in (with Jessie this time, just to be on the safe side!) and her response was: 'You cleared it up properly! Goodness me, the floors have seen worse than that and people don't usually do such a good job cleaning or even apologise!'

Strange how most dog tales are funnier in hindsight – but not that one! It still sends shivers down my spine. But I guess things like that happen when you're trying your hardest to please everyone. I didn't want to let the mother down, the PAT charity, Mike or myself, and most of all the patients. I can see now that I didn't need to put on the full therapy dog show – the dogs were already doing that job quite well for all to see. One little 'oopsie' from Leo (which was totally my fault) was not going to ruin everything. I just needed to take a deep breath, look at the bigger picture and remind myself I must learn to say no when the dog has signalled it is time to go. Something I have never forgotten ... and weirdly, it feels much easier now that I have that in the back of my mind.

17

Leo sharing the magic

AS MY DAYS VISITING WITH THE DOGS were getting busier and more frequent, I began to wonder how I was going to maintain this pace long-term.

Monty retired a short time after we were first invited onto paediatric oncology and met Alice Razza. He was fine and enjoyed meeting the young patients and getting all the cuddles, but I started to notice how tired he was at the end of a day on which he had done a visit and realised that the touch of arthritis we were managing with supplements was now beginning to slow him down. The day after a visit he seemed stiffer and I concluded that it was probably down to the hard corridor floors and the fact that it is quite some distance you cover walking around the hospital. Ethically, it was only fair to consider his retirement sooner rather than later, and besides, he still had an important role to play in my mission outside the hospital. He could still enjoy trotting into the care homes with Totty, I just thought it was unfair to ask any more of my faithful gentleman, the dog who always gave more than he took. I still had Leo and Jessie to shoulder the growing swell of hospital visit requests.

Usually, when one avenue of your life goes a little crazy, another decides to whirl you into the stratosphere too. And I remember that's exactly what happened through an entire eighteen months starting in the busy summer of 2014 ...

Jessie's puppies were just gorgeous – time-consuming too! Alex had looked after the pups while we were all together in France for thirty-six hours watching Harry compete in the rowing competition. Ten days later, once the pups had been weaned, Ollie and I headed to Florida, safe in the knowledge that Mike had taken leave so that he could look after the pups with help from Harry, who had now completed his rowing season. I felt confident with the arrangement and we had been through this a couple of times now, so everyone knew what to do. And there's no way that puppies can be anything but the priority as, in our home, the 'nursery' is in the middle of the kitchen. After spending every night with them in their first three weeks of life, making sure they and Jessie were feeding well, I missed them, but I think Mike and Harry were glad to get rid of me! Being so much in demand at the hospital put me in a 'need to be busy' zone, mixed with worry over my mum, who was ill after being diagnosed with cancer at the time, and being there for the boys' activities and everything else at home. It was all getting a bit mind fogging.

I was worried about my mum and didn't want these thoughts to get the better of me. Over the summer she spent almost six weeks in hospital, with a few of those nights in intensive care after becoming very unwell due to an adverse reaction to some chemotherapy. It was a truly awful time and of course, once she had made it out of hospital and home, she had a huge amount of recovery to do.

Throughout the summer, Leo and I visited a number of patients in the evenings, outside our normal daytime visits, and that suited everyone better to have the dogs to sit with and talk to when the rest of the hospital turned down its activities and switched into that quiet phase and the heavy feeling of a long night ahead.

At the end of that very eventful summer Mike was invited as the guest 'human doctor' to speak at the British Veterinary Orthopaedic Association conference in Brighton. He was invited to speak on developmental musculoskeletal conditions in children and saw it also as an opportunity to speak to the vets about picking up the symptoms of the discospondylitis (which in human beings is called osteomyelitis) that Leo had suffered the year before. Collaboration between human and animal doctors, the physicians and vets, the sharing of knowledge, could really benefit each other as the physiology and illnesses between animals and humans is much more closely related than many realise.

I can't help translating this in terms of the human-animal bond, because the more I witness how therapy dogs tune in to the needs of human beings, the more I realise how extraordinary the bond between the two species really is. To have my dogs' companionship while the pressure was on my family again at the time of my mum's awful illness made me very grateful. I really don't know, again, what I would have done without my dogs. The visits to the children to distract me from worrying about Mum were bonding us closer and closer, I could feel it happening. In particular, Leo and I were becoming a well-honed double act and I felt that I could trust him 100 per cent to deliver the smiles and the love. While Mike and the boys appreciate the physical presence of Monty, Totty, Jessie and Leo, I can see how I rely on them more for their emotional support and the unconditional love that they always have on tap. The same support that every patient we meet receives too.

Kim Sutton decided to ask if we could concentrate on the children from now on as that seemed to be where my dogs were making the biggest impression and bringing in the most astounding results. She was especially proud of the feedback received after visits to intensive care and oncology. She also knew I loved it and the number of visits I made in a week was growing. I had worked out a way of juggling my business, family and my volunteering role, fast becoming more than a hobby, and I was now visiting up to three times a week with one of my dogs. Leo's special gift with our young patients was improving their quality of life and changing people's minds about the new level of intervention being delivered by therapy dogs.

On every visit, I have the privilege of seeing the children's faces change from pain, boredom, frustration and all the other nouns and adjectives that cover how a child responds to an enforced period of hospitalisation. It's wonderful to see how the arrival of a dog can usually change their expression to one of delight in an instant.

* * *

It was Lewis Tupper's sixth birthday when he made one of his regular respite visits to Naomi House, the hospice near Winchester, where he was able to spend some quality time with his family. Leo was an old friend of Lewis's, having met him at the children's hospital when he had been in for long-term care due to his complex special needs and disabilities, and he loved Leo so much. I saw the boy light up when my dog appeared and, somehow, when they sat close to each other, Lewis's gentleness blended with Leo's calm to create a unique peace. That respite birthday was something Mum, Trish, Dad, Paul and Lewis's older brother Adam were able to enjoy with Lewis and I could see how Leo's presence acted as a kind of equaliser – a distraction that was common to all, even when he was sitting at his patient's side. If anyone was getting a bigger share of the attention, it was Leo!

Again, Leo shared his magic with the wider family, and as always, I was keen to support the sibling, because Adam loved Leo too. And, yes, I know where all this came from – Harry, because I know how he struggled when Ollie was in hospital. It's not easy for the sibling at home when all the attention must appear to be on the one in hospital. It's a balancing act with time, attention and distraction, so we were lucky to have the dogs at home. They were the one consistent source of attention that each one of us could rely on in our own way on that bumpy ride that we shared.

On the way home from that birthday visit to Lewis I thought of a friend who had asked me how I could smile after visiting poorly children and especially after visiting a hospice. I remember saying that it's 'how' you visit, because the smiles and the fun times override everything. You can create the most beautiful memories there, as anywhere, and that is what is so important to remember every time you step over the threshold: it's about them, never about you.

We saw Lewis several times in hospital, at his home and in the hospice. One time Leo was enjoying himself so much at the hospice, basking in all the fuss from several other patients and families that he refused to leave and I had to carry him out of the building! When that happens, everyone thinks it's hilarious, but Leo is really heavy. That day, to add insult to very near injury, he then refused to get in the car, so I had to lift him again ... that's Leo for you: an easy-going super-dog until you want him to do something he really does not want to do. I put it down to him being happy in his work and it's very likely that he gets the same buzz I do when we have a good visit. I know there are times when I would like to stay longer too. It's a good, soul-deep feeling of connection that you don't want to let go of. But I must remember the ethics of working with a dog and that my other dogs (and humans) are waiting at home for me, so it's often on the drive home that I allow myself to enjoy the feeling attached to a good visit – the feeling that something good happened and you want to experience it again and again. It's very addictive and always a pleasure to visit, never a chore.

We were there for James Lewis too when he needed Leo most to brighten his eleven-week stay in hospital, following the insertion of a Hickman line (a hollow catheter) in his chest. When Leo met James, he was waiting for his heart transplant. He was on intravenous support in UHS for heart failure and later went on to have his heart transplant at the Freeman Hospital, Newcastle upon Tyne. Hospitals are scary places, particularly for children, and the build-up and preparation for surgery is an alien process. I can only imagine how very scary a prospect this must have been at that time for the entire family, who knew more about what it all entailed than James himself. The list of procedures to follow was to become part of this boy's life and the accompanying weeks in hospital, when Leo and the rest of the dogs became welcome visitors to brighten the long days.

That's why, when we met James again when he was eight years old and I spoke to his mum while he was in PICU, we were convinced that trusting in Leo's calm and his warmth would reduce James's anxiety before he went into theatre. By this stage, James knew all about what to expect and that's why he was so anxious about being anaesthetised. To have that short time with Leo, sitting with him, stroking him, I wondered if James could feel the dog's good steady heartbeat against the palm of his hand. Even though he was intubated at the time, he looked relaxed, stroking Leo's big, warm chest.

With Leo a regular visitor when James was at SCH, a friendship and a trust developed that brought us very close to the family. James's mum very kindly wrote:

> 'For us as parents, having Lyndsey to talk to, who is so kind and empathetic, always a listening ear, was really helpful. We too enjoyed stroking Leo and friends over the years. For vulnerable children who are feeling unwell or traumatised from their medical

journeys, it is really beneficial to spend time with a lovely dog who just gives cuddles and unconditional love.'

As I've said many times before, the work we do is a privilege. If my 'indoor dog walk' has given a patient and their family some comfort then I am the beneficiary just as much as they are.

18

Right place, right time

UNTIL I STARTED VOLUNTEERING with Animal Assisted Intervention (AAI) I had never really thought through the number of situations and conditions where a therapy dog could definitely be the bridge between a patient and the treatment provided by a clinical team. It turns out, I didn't need to think or over-plan because once the word was out, the cases came to us.

Sometimes we are just there at the right time, like the day we met a young girl in her room on the medical ward. Her mother asked if I could nip in and see her daughter, who was sitting on a thick mat on the floor playing with some toys. I never like to say the word 'no' to children and on this occasion, we were at the beginning of our visit so we had the time. I knelt down to sit on the floor beside the mat, we said our hellos, were chatting and Leo was getting lots of fuss, and then the child suddenly had an epileptic fit. I was closest to her so with one hand through the handle on the dog's lead, I was able to catch her head before it reached the ground. Leo didn't move, not a whisker. He stayed steady as a rock as his patient carried on trying to stroke him while making involuntary movements ... she didn't let go of his coat. Her mother had seen her fit like that many times but not maintain the hold on anything the way she held Leo.

The nursing staff and her mother monitored the fit and I must admit I would have felt completely out of my depth had I been there alone. But then I would never be alone with a patient, such is the guidance for our visits. There is always a parent or member of staff close by and I am thankful for that support.

So many conditions and disorders are invisible, silent killers and children are just as likely to be held in their grasp as adults. I recall a patient who came to us through the child and adolescent mental health service (CAMHS). This patient, like many young people who find themselves weaving through a mental health issue, felt isolated, confused, and sometimes their behaviour can be confusing to the adults around them – but not to dogs.

No two cases are the same and I didn't think Leo would meet anyone who could hug him too much, but this particular patient came close. The girl was 15 years old and had reached the point where all she needed was an end to her wait for a bed in a unit that treated eating disorders. Angry, clearly exhausted by both her illness and the route that saw her admitted to the children's hospital rather than direct to the eating disorders unit, she had turned her body to the wall. The nurse who asked if I could visit told me she was not at all happy and really didn't want to talk to anyone, especially the nurses. 'She may well swear at you,' she warned! I knew the nurse was there behind me as I opened the door and I knew what she was expecting to hear, and so it came: 'F**k off!'

I was ready for it: 'Well, I can if you want me to but my name is Lyndsey and I am not part of the medical team. I am a hospital volunteer with a therapy dog if you would like to see him ... Up to you, yes or no?' The girl turned, saw Leo's head peeping round the door frame into her room and said: 'Oh, you can come in, but I don't want any more nurses!' And so, under the watchful eye of a mental health nurse observing through the door, we walked into the room.

The girl turned towards us, still sitting in the corner of the room on a pillow on the floor, with her long pyjama trousers failing to disguise the thinness of her crossed legs. I could see that Leo was visibly concerned for her. His entire body language was telling me that he wanted to get closer to her, almost desperate to gently approach her. And then she held out her hand to Leo, so thin and shaking, and he sat close beside her. That was all the cue she needed to throw her arms around him and calmly he lay down and rested his head in her lap. She said nothing as I sat with them and left Leo to do what he felt he needed, to comfort this girl who had started our visit so inauspiciously.

Finally, she found her voice and quietly began to talk to me about the future. I think she saw this as her chance to share with someone, totally independent, in confidence, and she eased into it with her eyes constantly on Leo. She was angry that, after many months in the grip of her eating disorder and finally making the decision that she was ready for treatment, there now wasn't a bed in the right unit. I said to her that she was on the pathway now and once she had her bed in the specialist unit, the likelihood was that someone else would be hugging Leo as they waited for a bed there too.

'Very true,' she said and then she started to cry. She cuddled Leo and cried some more. She cried so much, I thought that Leo would drown in tears. The top of his head was wet, it still felt damp when we got home. The girl was to be our last visit of the day and I was glad because Leo was emotionally exhausted.

He was there for his patient, in the moment, and it was because he was present for her that the girl communicated with me through him. She leant on him, physically and emotionally. It was tough to watch this brave girl in such turmoil but at the same time what I was seeing fired my need to find out more about this bond, this invisible link that has the ability for patients to start to talk and to find their way to heal.

Having been unsuccessful in her first nomination, volunteer manager Kim Sutton set about compiling a new PAT Dog of the Year nomination for 2015. I was over the moon because we were then three years into my mission, my promise to myself, and because Leo was truly loving his celebrity status. After our first nomination I decided to launch a Facebook page called 'Leo & Friends Therapy Dogs' just to let people know what we were all about and thinking that it would encourage patients to share their stories and some of the hundreds of pictures taken with Leo or any of my dogs during our visits.

The page was named 'Leo & Friends', mirrored in the title of this book, because this all came at a special time for me, Leo and the team. The name felt right because I'm sure Leo felt like he was the 'top dog' of my team but, in truth, all my dogs were very important to my mission in their own way. The thing is, I soon had a fit of the jitters with the Facebook idea, deciding it was a bit arrogant and convincing myself that it made me look like a show-off. So, I switched it off and kept it private and hidden! But by the time of the second nomination, I decided that it was time to cast off self-doubt, or whatever it was that was holding me back, and go for it.

It still took a parent at the hospital asking me if I shared any of what we do on social media to convince me that it was a good thing to do. He said that I should, in his words: '... shout about this, shout about the brilliant work you do with your therapy dogs. Thank you so much!' Right after that conversation I went home and, with some trepidation, activated the page. Within hours we were counting the 'likes'.

I was very fortunate to have the incredibly talented Daniel Howarth's illustration of Leo wearing a stethoscope to use on the page by then, and as soon as it was live again, I couldn't understand why I'd held back before. The whole thing took off at pace and parents joined in, posting their stories to the page, which made me feel so proud of 'Leo & Friends'. And when we could announce that we had made it to the final line-up of PAT Dog of the Year, the media waggons rolled back in! This time around, I was ready for them.

I began to think of all our patients and angel patients who had known us. I thought of little Archie Adams smiling when he saw his hand resting on Leo's paw: it didn't matter that he couldn't feel it because he could see it. And I remembered the tweet from the hospital confirming how the staff had seen his vital signs improve. I thought of a teenage lad, who we supported ahead of his surgery. Leo sat with him on the day ward as I spoke to him about anything other than medical matters to help with his anxiety. It was easy to think of so many more young patients who would remember Leo helping them in their moment of fear. And there was the growing pile of thank you letters from parents telling me how they felt about 'Leo & Friends', how extraordinary they were and how much pleasure the dogs gave and, most precious of all, how they gave hope.

My blood rushing with excitement and my head filled with ideas, I had stickers produced from Daniel's drawing and an additional design with all four of my dogs in PAT uniform sitting in a row with the strapline: 'One of these dogs made me smile today'. The children loved the stickers and they could now choose which one they wanted to take with them, whether they were off on a transfer to another hospital or going home. Some of my friends didn't get it, any of it, and I'm not sure that some of my extended family understood me either. But Mike got it, he gets me, and once he'd seen Leo working with the children in his hospital, he started to speak to me about even more patients he thought could benefit from the dogs' support, especially those who he knew would be in for a long while. Suddenly, and amazingly, I felt that I was a small part of the clinical team, too.

One of my most treasured possessions, to this day, is the lanyard from the children's hospital that the then senior matron, Kate Pye, gave to me. I could have hugged her – she could never have known how honoured I felt to have that around my neck. To me, that piece of fabric in a rainbow of colours with the words 'Southampton Children's Hospital' said that I belonged. The timing of that lanyard's arrival couldn't have been better. I was feeling pulled in all directions and the exposure of all our good work in the media had, sadly, encouraged a few critics out of the woodwork too.

There's always a danger in doing something well that benefits others – you can make it look so easy that everyone thinks they want to join you. In some ways we were verging on being the victims of our own success. The truth of the matter is not every dog has the qualities to be a PAT dog and not every dog can work with every kind of patient. Just as Leo is better with children than the elderly. So began a tricky time when suddenly it seemed everyone wanted to work with children, without perhaps realising that taking a therapy dog into hospitals, hospices, care homes or schools needs to be overseen to get it right for the patients. A handler is only as effective as the dog on the end of the lead. When nursing staff and parents reported that they felt some of the dogs turning up on the children's wards were not suited to paediatric patients I was worried. But it turned out they weren't talking about mine. I wasn't in charge of the volunteers and often had no clue who they were talking about, but suddenly I was being asked why these people were turning up. Suffice to say, it was awkward but I wasn't about to let it threaten what I had started to create and what was valued by the paediatric healthcare teams.

In addition, there were difficulties with timings. It turned out that patients were reluctant to go home on discharge because they were 'waiting to see the dog' that they had heard visited on a Tuesday afternoon! OMG, my dogs had turned into bed blockers! I was mortified, so immediately decided to vary all of my visiting days to make it right. I started to wonder why doing a voluntary role that I loved was becoming so tricky. This already awkward time was later topped off by the appearance of an animal rights activist in the hospital car park!

I was patient, I listened to the critic telling me that my dog was being used for my personal gain and was potentially unhappy in his role. The final irony was that when the lady finished saying her piece, Leo refused to move. I turned around as if I was heading back into the hospital and said: 'Come on then', which seemed to do the trick – he stood up and walked back towards the entrance ready to start visiting all over again. He loves it! I smiled inside: 'Good lad,' I thought to myself.

When I started volunteer visiting with Leo, I realised that both he and I would make more of a difference if we spent our weekends at the hospital where he was happy, not at dog shows or in the showring, which has never been his thing. When my mind drifts to possibly trying him there again, as a veteran, I hold the thought because I suspect Leo's sentiments will remain: 'What am I doing here, boss, and where are the children?'

Leo is always at his happiest in the hospital, with children – and I'm at my happiest right beside him. It was so frustrating being in this position and having to defend the work of the therapy dogs: how they enjoy being fussed over and loved by the children, staff and parents in the hospital, and when off-duty, they enjoyed lovely long walks and time at home with their family. Then I realised that I needed to see this opportunity as a positive – turn it around and use it to re-enforce the all-important message that taking therapy dogs into an establishment is controlled and overseen. It's just the dogs who make it look so easy.

I will admit that there were times in the autumn of 2015 when I felt like quitting. It wasn't in the face of a bit of criticism, it was a culmination of factors, which included people who didn't understand what I was doing or why. I knew the reason why I was volunteering and that's all that mattered, so I shook it off. When I was tired or feeling a little bit low, overwhelm, frustration and sadness, all my old enemies, were on my back. I occasionally returned to familiar ground of anxiety and was sometimes worried about the onset of another bout of self-doubt, which didn't feel good at all. I thought how difficult it was for parents sitting for hours and hours at their children's bedside. How bad it was for them and how much joy and hope the dogs brought into those shadowy times. If it hadn't been for that and all the PAT Dog of the Year finalist commitments, I may well have stopped right then but ... What on earth was I thinking?

I was back in an environment where I felt comfortable and confident – healthcare gave me a buzz when I was working in paid employment in a hospital in my twenties and now working in a voluntary role with my therapy dogs put me on a pretty much permanent high. And, biggest recognition of all, I had been given the Southampton Children's Hospital lanyard by Kate Pye. I belonged. We also now had SCH livery for the dogs so that those welcome on the children's wards could be recognised apart from those who were general PAT dogs and this had helped alleviate the concerns of the staff who wanted to request my team. With Leo or Jessie at my side, we were making changes for the better. We were giving patients and parents something genuinely good and supportive that simply hadn't been there when Ollie was on the Piam Brown oncology ward seven years earlier.

This was not a time to give up – it was a time to get going! Besides, I couldn't let Leo down, or our patients, such as 'Gorgeous George' O'Shaughnessy, his mum, dad or his sister Bella.

George was just coming up to his second birthday when he met Leo for the first time on the Piam Brown children's cancer ward. It was towards the end of 2014 when he was diagnosed with acute lymphoblastic leukaemia and although he didn't speak much for his age, seeing Leo and the others made him really excited, so every visit we were met with lots of pointing, smiling and George encouraging the dogs over to him, and of course they were more than happy to oblige. Leo quickly became George's best mate and while the dog enjoyed all the strokes on offer, I took the opportunity to see how George's mum, Amy, was feeling on those days with long gaps when nothing really happened.

I guessed that our journey with George and his family would be long and a little bit rocky because that's leukaemia, and true enough, over the next five years our visits became more regular and we were staying longer. According to Amy, Leo and his friends became the highlight of those quiet hospital days. As soon as he saw a dog on the ward, George headed straight for them. He enjoyed giving lots of fuss and strokes. He loved playing 'Who did that?' – when I covered the dog's eyes and George stroked Leo, pretending Leo wouldn't know who it was. George always laughed so hard in that time of his new and difficult normal during a hospital stay, especially when Bella was visiting. His sister loved the dogs too. The children had the biggest smiles on their faces and the family were able to take lots of photos – all with a smiling dog in the shot!

I realised that we were needed in so many places and I worried that the patients weren't getting the best of what we could offer. I was feeling the weight of responsibility, but it was a good weight and not a burden, and I still believe that it's a weight I am meant to carry. The thing was, the more I did, the more there seemed to be to do and was there enough of me to go round? I was one woman with four dogs receiving a huge number of requests to visit. The round trip to the hospital and back would routinely take up to four hours by the time I had prepped the dog, driven there, parked, signed in, carried out perhaps a ninety-minute visit, taken twenty minutes to navigate the public, who wanted to say hello en route in or out, and then driven home … and that's before you count the time spent preparing whichever dog to ensure they were super-clean! Something had to give.

At the same time, all that reading about the human-animal bond had thrown up more and more links to dogs involved in Animal Assisted Intervention. Was this something I could study?

I googled and swept through Amazon and everywhere on the internet that could tell me more and point me in the right direction of books, courses and qualifications. There had been a course running in the UK but it had been pulled. I searched harder and found one in the States – Denver University. Perfect! But I didn't have the qualifications. Now what had seemed a great idea to leave school in the middle of my A-levels and skip university didn't seem so great after all.

The only thing that kept my anger and disappointment at bay was visiting the hospital, and as there was so much to do there, so many requests for my dogs, it proved the almost perfect distraction. I could sort all of these demands. Quitting was not an option and not my style. I just needed to refocus on who and where I was visiting. I could do that after I had kept my promise to Ollie and returned to volunteer at Give Kids the World in America, this time just before Christmas 2015.

The seed of study had been planted; all I needed to do was find a way to make it happen. And that's when fate, and America, took a hand.

19

All the way to America …

DRIVING IN FLORIDA, WITH OLLIE IN THE CAR, I was lost and totally out of my comfort zone. This was our third trip to Give Kids the World and my second as a volunteer alongside Ollie and, although I'm not keen on the drive from the airport, I just love it when we get to the resort. As soon as we arrive, I always end up shedding a tear. It really is the most magical place on earth, with the most incredibly inspiring people who share a poignant common bond – children who have survived or are coping with a life-threatening or life-limiting illness.

To the blissfully uninitiated it may sound like the last place anyone would go for a laugh and a genuinely good time, but thinking that would be wrong. One way or another, everyone there has much to celebrate in life, despite at times enduring pain and loss. It really is a place that shows the importance of enjoying our loved ones, living life to its fullest, and the incredible, never to be underestimated power of empathy and kindness.

They say if you want to know what someone needs, then walk a mile in their shoes. All the families visiting GKTW have walked those miles and I'm sure it's the reason why I feel so much empathy for the parents I meet when I visit the children at SCH. I recognise the common signs: the long, slightly vague stare, the confusion, the occasional tears and anger, but I don't know how they feel, because no one can truly know to what degree someone feels pain. What you do know, for absolute certainty, is that they have periods where they are hurting inside, they are lost, confused, they don't want to be there and they just want to be able to take their child home.

Wrestling with a bunch of emotions that usually appear in isolation, or alongside grief over the loss of your previous relatively carefree life and shock, which all settles in a knot in the pit of your stomach or gets stuck in your chest. You can't move it, but a distraction of the kind and respectful variety will ease its grip – just for a while – helps you see things differently, maybe just a little clearer, if only for a few moments in time. I know ... because I have been there.

The timing of this trip could not have been more perfect, although it had been planned for months, way before I began to feel the self-induced pressure of being pulled in all directions. I needed to be there. It was lovely to hear Harry, who by then was 18 and in his first year at university, say the same thing about GKTW, that it answered the need for reconnecting the family after a period in his life where his sibling was ill and his parents were juggling everything. Every time I go there, I feel that I belong and just walking through the gates is like being embraced by a loved one who will never judge you, never share your secrets and never, ever let you down.

In that way, I think, there are huge similarities with the human-animal bond. There is almost an unspoken understanding. In a way animal companionship has the edge over a human relationship because everything is communicated without speech. Yes, I talk to my dogs all the time, but they don't utter a word back to me. The many times I've looked into Monty's eyes and seen total understanding; he knew exactly when to offer a paw for extra support. And Leo 'the leaner' is the main man when it comes to well-timed cuddle-ups. I don't have to say a word and genuine unconditional love is there for me. Not a single verbal request is required in this calm, silent communication. No wonder we feel the human-animal bond so strongly.

Maybe that's why, even though I'm married to a surgeon, I have huge respect for veterinary surgeons because their patients can't verbalise where it hurts or how they feel. It would be really handy if they could, but because they can't, a vet has to rely entirely on their knowledge, experience, skill, powers of observation and intuition to reach a diagnosis. It's a lot to ask and a great deal rests on their expertise.

We look for and then establish ways of understanding and communicating with our animal companions that don't require them to answer us back. Dogs, over thousands of years of domestication, have developed a way of giving us what they feel (or perhaps have learnt) that we need. And, in general, I think they do it perfectly and effortlessly because they like to please us. If there's a reward in there somewhere then fine. Everyone's happy! Monty, Totty, Jessie and Leo could have 'people-pleaser' as a second name. That's why Leo, my king of the people-pleasers, is such a good therapy dog. He seems to key into what his patients want and need from him. He gives that generously and wholeheartedly without expecting anything in return. Children who can't speak, move, touch, smile, find a way of reaching Leo. Despite their being in an alien environment and potentially experiencing pain, confusion, fear, despair, they reach out, to stroke him and touch his warm fur. And they find it there. That's the power of connection.

I had already read *The Power of Wagging Tails* by Dr Dawn A. Marcus and I intended to look through Dr Aubrey Fine's *Handbook on Animal-Assisted Therapy* during the ten-hour flight to Florida. I packed a few more books into my suitcase so that I could make the best of the time away from the normal routine of things at home to read and increase my knowledge. As far as I could tell from my reading so far, Leo had played his part in assisting patients like Becky, Alice and Jo. But I realised there was more to this that we could be doing at SCH.

My head was buzzing with ideas – but first I had to find a course where you didn't need a degree to enrol. I was still kicking myself for not sticking with my A-levels and having to play catch-up, especially now I was in my late forties. But how far was regret going to take me? Besides, if I had continued in higher education and taken a different path I would never have worked in healthcare, most likely never met Mike, and definitely never have had my sons, the life or dogs I had and loved. There was no place for regrets and besides, how ironic was it that I was heading for the USA, one location in the world where Animal Assisted Intervention is more widely adopted in healthcare facilities as part of human therapy and recovery?

After our volunteer shifts at GKTW, Ollie and I returned to our rental house and every evening, I read or revisited the University of Denver's website and wished I had that degree needed for the Animals and Human Health course. The frustration was driving me nuts! Why didn't I just call them? After all, I was in the USA and in a relatively similar time zone. I plucked up courage and called the Institute for Human-Animal Connection (IHAC) at the university. As luck would have it, I spoke to a lady called Marla, who said: 'Oh, that's OK. I don't have those qualifications either but I studied as a Pet Partners handler [a large charity which provides volunteers and therapy dogs in the USA] with years of experience ... just like you.'

She told me that I might be able to enrol on the Animals and Human Health course and could study as a distance learner, which ultimately meant a commitment of 350 contact hours plus lots of background reading and writing between January and November, so almost all of 2016.

Hope was more than alive.

I put the phone down and carried on reading. I could discuss the cost and time commitment with Mike when he arrived in Florida with Harry to join us for our Christmas break. I felt sure he would agree that it was the right thing to do.

And I was right. By the time I landed back in the UK fresh from the family break and was back with the dogs, I was filled with the special energy that only GKTW provides;

I was ready to email Marla, this time to enrol on the course. The thing is, as you're probably aware by now, I'm a fixer – driven to fix!

Once I had taken the plunge and spoken to Marla on the phone, I knew this dream of mine was possible. The commitment was heavy but I convinced myself that I could manage. I wasn't quite sure how but I had time to work that out and besides, there is always a way when you want to do something that means so much. The course start date was less than three weeks away, starting at the end of January (2016), so how could I possibly increase the hours I was visiting with the dogs? After all, I was already feeling the overwhelm before I left for Florida. I decided to permanently sideline the visits to care homes, safe in the knowledge that other PAT dogs in the area could visit those and I wouldn't be letting the residents down. Decision made, I felt I could focus on my course and the paediatric patients at the hospital.

After New Year, everything happened so quickly. My acceptance for the course came through; the next thing I knew I was wrestling with the university's teaching software and feeling a bit stupid and embarrassed but genuinely excited too. Marla was incredibly patient with me and told me that my experience as a handler was very similar to hers, which gave me a helping of confidence which I felt I needed to step into this arena. In no time at all I was up to speed with the technology and loving every minute of the course, which was pretty full-on from the start.

I was busy doing modules, taking part in discussions, reading like crazy and writing essays throughout the first couple of months, and I was loving it. It was great for me being in a time zone ahead of the rest of the cohort – my submissions were never late! If it was a noon deadline in Denver, it was mid-afternoon for some of them in different states and 7pm for me. Initially there were ten of us starting the course but over time that number reduced to seven. Unsurprisingly, I was the only one from 'across the pond' and the only one who was just a dog handler.

I admit that, at first, I found it quite intimidating being surrounded by social workers, psychology graduates and other healthcare professionals, but it didn't take long for me to realise that I had plenty to contribute to the group from a wide range of experiences, including four years of working with therapy dogs in the same kind of environments. Some in the group aspired to work as therapists mostly with dogs or horses, but not everyone had pets and some had no experience of working alongside an animal at all.

Two of the students worked directly with children, but the one whose work was most closely related to mine was Amy, who worked as a Child Life Specialist at Cincinnati Children's Hospital Medical Center. We got on from the start and we are still in contact occasionally as we have so much in common. Amy's role is very similar to our play specialists in the UK, so we worked well together on collaborative projects and loved drawing on each other's experiences. I was like a sponge soaking up all the information shared by my fellow students and I learnt from them all but especially anyone working with children. However, I wasn't prepared for all I heard.

Some of the scenarios shared on the course were very distressing and that opened my eyes to how AAI fitted into the broader aspects of working in paediatrics. One of the students worked with children, some of whom had suffered psychological trauma, and her discussions in the modules were both shocking and inspiring; she was always careful never to break confidentiality of a particular case and just described generalised scenarios. Within just the first few weeks of study I realised that what I was doing at SCH was such a small part of what was achievable working with therapy dogs. My mind was racing even before they mentioned the possibility of attending the annual conference, scheduled for May 2016.

It was around March when the university began promoting the Institute for Human Animal Connection conference. They chose 'Animals on the Mind' as the headline and I was not required to attend as part of my course, especially given that I lived almost five thousand miles away. But when I heard that most of my study group were thinking of going, I was not going to be left out. It was only the Atlantic Ocean between us after all! I decided it would be brilliant to fly over, attend the meeting and meet everyone in the flesh. Besides, the speakers looked really interesting and we were told there would be some special dogs attending too! I didn't need any more good reasons to convince me that I must make that journey.

I set off on the thirteen-hour flight alone, with a hire car booked for the other end. As the plane took off, I wondered how I had become so determined to do something that required me to fly thousands of miles and this time hire a car without even Ollie to stop me panicking if I got lost! I am 100 per cent sure I wouldn't have done it if I hadn't felt so passionate about this course; this was the way forward and the perfect fit for me. I was devouring the course information and my brain was on high alert with ideas popping into my head all the time. The more I learned, the more I wanted to.

Without a shadow of a doubt, this course was going to be the best fiftieth birthday present to myself EVER!

Of course, while I had my eyes glued to a computer screen or stuck in a book, my mind was still on organising the visits to our patients in the hospital and the dogs still had to be fed, walked and washed. Our family still had to function and so did my business. Normal life had to be fitted around my studies and I would be a very big liar if I said that it was easy. I had successfully managed to put another layer of work and angst into the mix and, once again, something had to give because I could not stretch another second out of my days.

The good difference about this bout of overwhelm was that it didn't bring the dark thoughts – because I could see light at the end of the tunnel. All I needed to do was get a little more organised and, if I could, arrange some help.

Part Three:

Welcome to the Rollercoaster

20
Teamwork

MY DOGS ARE MY FAMILY, so I'm always thorough when I do my new-home checks. I need to be absolutely sure my offspring are going to great homes where good people will look after them properly and love them dearly. One of the pups in Totty's final litter was very calm and cuddly and, I thought, would be perfect for an elderly lady and her bachelor son, who were both happy to be home for the pup and physically able to walk him and do everything else that goes with setting up for a new 'baby' in the house. We had chatted a lot on the phone and they had visited twice to see the pups with Totty and taken the opportunity to ask lots of questions. I was convinced that the little one was going to a good home. Also, they had been on my puppy waiting list since I'd met the lady eighteen months before, so it was their turn and I thought I had the perfect pup for them.

The handover went well and everyone seemed happy, but three weeks later, I received a call to say that having a puppy was not right for them after all. Things had changed for the lady since she'd joined my waiting list and, as she hadn't declared them before, I admit to feeling angry and, most of all, overwhelming guilt for getting it so wrong for the pup. I am grateful that they called me and I could collect him, bring him home and start again. These things happen – but not normally to me. This pup was not going to be let down twice ...

Once he was back home, snuggling back with Totty and the rest of my pack, I realised again how lovely this little pup was and how much I wanted to keep him! I was under pressure, because I had promised myself that I wouldn't be tempted to keep one this time as the boys had A-levels and GCSEs looming and I had quite enough on my plate with my volunteering, four dogs and my business. As the puppy was only just back home, I didn't want to leave him that afternoon so I took him to the hairdresser's with me, where he was so incredibly calm and so gorgeous, greeting everyone as if he owned the place – and he was still under 12 weeks old. I looked at him with huge pride as everyone fussed over him and he lapped up the attention in spades. 'He's a mini-Leo!' I couldn't help saying it out loud. Little Archie, that's what we called him, was the image of his dad and so I knew that whoever I was to choose to have this pup as their companion had to be someone very special indeed – otherwise he was staying home with me whatever the rest of the family might think!

I happened to include a picture of Archie making his debut at the hairdresser's on one of my personal Facebook posts and when my friend Karen saw it, she called me to find out what had happened and to ask if she could come over for a puppy cuddle. Karen and her husband, Alastair, fell in love with Archie at first sight and hoped that I would be able to part with him. So, Archie joined the Ramsay household, which included their other golden retriever, Hattie, and I couldn't have been happier. What a relief to see those two pups I'd bred in their garden together, adoring each other from the first minute! I had the best of every option: I could keep my promise not to keep a pup and Archie had a fabulous new home and I could see him whenever I saw my friends. Perfect!

It wasn't long before Karen was telling me how wonderful Archie was with the children at West Hill Park school, where her husband was head teacher. In fact, he was so wonderful that she was going to make his position official as she had some time when she could volunteer alongside him. When he was old enough, Archie qualified with Pets As Therapy and became the school's first therapy dog, with over three hundred children to give him attention.

Then I had an idea. If Archie was so good with children, how would Karen feel about joining me visiting the children in SCH? Karen was well aware what I did at the hospital with Leo, and after spending lots of time with us and meeting some of the clinical team I had been working with, she saw how valuable her contribution could be. Joining with Archie for the meet-and-greet sessions would be similar to what they were doing at the school. Then taking one step further as an observer, she saw the Animal Assisted Therapy being achieved with Felix after his terrible accident, which included helping him with his physiotherapy – and that was it. She wanted to be part of it. Karen and Archie joined me in April 2016 and a few months later, Karen's daughter, Hannah, qualified their other dog Hattie to join us. We were a team.

I can't emphasise enough the value of good friends. Having Karen and Hannah's help meant that we could cover requests from the wards, which, in turn, freed up some time for me and my studies – including giving me the time to travel to Denver. Phew!

Just before I flew out to attend the conference in May, I took a call from Marla, who had been looking at our 'Leo & Friends' Facebook page and saw pictures of Leo with Felix and baby Archie. She wondered if I could give her permission to use a couple of the pictures as part of the IHAC marketing campaign. I was taken aback by the request and totally chuffed, especially when both sets of parents gave permission to send the large image files over to the university. I had nothing more to do, other than pack a bag, my laptop and more books, and head for Denver.

Reading on the plane put me in the mood for the conference, but I didn't need to cram in any study time as I was up to date with everything. It was just that I was in such a 'must study' mood that I could not give myself a break.

The next morning, after a good sleep, I drove across to the university in beautiful May sunshine, with views to the Colorado mountain tops, still snow-covered, in the distance. On arrival, I parked up and started walking across the campus to the meeting room where we were all due to gather for the meet-and-greet. I had never been part of a university before. Me, the school leaver who went straight to work. It felt incredible, I was in Denver and this was where I was studying. I had to stop, breathe and let that sink in. I knew it wouldn't be the kind of meet-and-greet that I was used to with a dog at my heel and so I was a little nervous about meeting everyone, but the second I walked into the foyer, I was faced with some familiar faces – on a huge banner there was Leo, Felix and his physiotherapy team. I beamed with joy and surprise – I felt my face light up. To me it was a sign that despite my anxiety, I belonged there. Our team was in the foyer!

I signed in, collected a delegate bag, and headed into the conference hall, where Marla came over to introduce herself. It was great to meet her after all the calls and online conversations over the past six months and she was as lovely as I had imagined. I went to sit with everyone from the cohort and all the 'guest' dogs at the front of the audience and took a deep breath. In that setting, with my new colleagues around me, I soon relaxed into a huge sense of belonging, which of course was helped by the assistance and therapy dogs who were part of the conference and lying at our feet. Added to that, I felt that I was within an auditorium of 'my people' and that feeling was about to get so much stronger. I opened the delegate pack and pulled out the leaflets … and there, in the listing of IHAC courses, was a photo of Leo with baby Archie in paediatric intensive care! Another slice of what I was doing, as my hobby at home was right there in Denver. I felt I could afford to relax some more.

The presentations were so inspiring, heart-rending, fascinating and extremely emotional. Tears flowed at the end of the presentation from Warrior Canine Connection, the American charity founded by and existing for veterans to provide them with support and assistance dogs. The stories made me cry unashamedly and once again I had my ideas head on. I wondered how I could get involved in some way or replicate this in the UK. My head was like a box of lit fireworks again but I had to cool it down because I needed all my brain cells to get through the course. I parked the idea and my enthusiasm but had a feeling that it would be back in my head at some point.

At the end of day one I had the honour of meeting author Dr Aubrey Fine, whose *Handbook on Assisted Animal Therapy* had been my reading on and off for the past year. I had taken my copy with me in case I had time between presentations to read, but of course I hadn't accounted for the fact that now I was with my student colleagues any time between lectures would be spent chatting! At the end of his presentation, I was glad I had the book with me – I couldn't resist talking to Dr Fine and ended up asking him for a photo and to sign my copy of his book. I treasure the words he wrote because he is so right:

> To Lyndsey, it was wonderful to meet you. I hope we will stay in touch. Always remember, animals bless our lives. Celebrate and cherish the bond! My best, Aubrey.

I spent six full days in Denver. The conference took up a couple of them and we had a gala dinner on the evening of the first day, an impressive event attended by most of the three hundred delegates. The IHAC had also arranged a selection of visits, one of them being a visit to the Kong factory to meet the creator of the Kong dog toy. A tour of the factory seeing how they were made was very interesting but the treat of the trip was meeting the office dogs who double as the testing team for new products!

For me, one of the huge pleasures of those six days away was meeting Ann Howie, clinical social worker and founder of Human-Animal Solutions, who was one of the lecturers for some of the courses at IHAC but not one of our main tutors despite being the author of various books on our reading list. Ann is incredibly passionate about AAI, so we immediately sparked up a conversation, but as these things go, there just wasn't enough time to really talk, so I marked her down for an email on my return home. I really got the feeling that Ann, with all her experience, would be the perfect person to talk to when this was over and I needed to filter some ideas. I already had her books, *Teaming with Your Therapy Dog* and *The Handler Factor*, as they were part of our book list, but I knew I wanted to ask more!

It was thanks to Marla that a visit to Colorado Children's Hospital was made possible for me to meet their volunteer manager and then shadow one of their 'Prescription Pets' handlers. I was expecting an inspirational day and I was not disappointed. Experiencing that the way the handlers there were partnering their therapy dogs was not that different to the service I had evolved at Southampton was really satisfying. One of their child patients was severely disabled and had lots of special needs, he reminded me of Lewis Tupper back home: somehow that boy found a fragment of energy from somewhere to want to try to reach out towards the therapy dog.

It was odd watching someone else do what I do, with a different dog and a slightly different approach but nevertheless a moment of the human-animal bond at work. But it was also wonderful to see some of the things they did, such as giving a card to every child to verify the team that had visited. Of course, they may have done that in case the hospital needed to apply a cost for the visit, but I knew we could adapt those cards for our free service at SCH – and there came the inspiration for the 'Top Trumps' style cards we now use. I created ours to have a mini biography of the dog, including some fun facts, on the front and images of them at work and play on the back. Each child is given one and the children in hospital for a while collect them. They are a useful discussion point not only for us but for the next shift of staff who arrive long after we have gone, as they can then strike up a conversation knowing their patient has seen whichever dog is pictured.

Within a blink of an eye, I was back home and back into the normal routine, but this time I had team colleagues to share the load and that was brilliant! I could cast off some of the guilt I felt at not being available to visit as much as I had before; before they started, I'd been visiting up to four times a week. However, after Denver, I was desperate to get back in there and start looking at everything with my new, inspired AAI hat on, blending all those influences with all that we were achieving at SCH. I was looking to change things but Jessie, bless her, quickly reminded me that some things never change ...

It was Jessie's turn for visiting day, giving Leo a rest as he had become my go-to dog for visiting children with planned AAI work. This was only because Leo was gentle and loved lingering, longer attention whereas Jessie, as I've explained, was a little more 'let's get on with it', which is great for the meet-and-greet which takes up approximately 75 per cent of our time in the hospital. Jessie is also good for meeting children who could be regarded as challenging. While Leo is likely to back away from a 'shouty' person, wondering what on earth he has done to deserve it, Jessie will stand squarely and inquisitively in a non-aggressive way with her mouth open as if smiling and just keep wagging her tail with a look of: 'Well, you can do that if you like but I'll be right here!' Jessie always knows what she wants.

While we waited on the ground floor for a lift to the children's wards at the top of the hospital, Jessie was all swishy tail wags and smiles for everyone passing, including the family standing beside us. I checked they were happy for us to travel up with them – something I always do – and we were given the go-ahead, which was good because the little girl, aged about three, was really enjoying stroking Jessie and my dog was clearly very keen on her. We got into the lift and the mother passed the girl a large bag of crisps that the family had been sharing. I had seen it on top of the pram, tucked into the folds of the hood. Now we had the ideal combination for Jessie – a small child holding a large bag of crisps in one hand and the other free and stroking a very adorable dog. Inside, I marvelled at the way my dog was being so good and we watched as the little one rested her head on Jessie's back as she very sweetly declared: 'I wuv you, Jessie!' And then I looked up to say how sweet that is to the parents and immediately heard: 'Crunch!' My crafty dog had been working her nose into the bag of crisps, which was in the girl's left hand. OMG, the shame! Everyone was laughing – except me. All I could do was apologise and offer to replace the crisps but the mother insisted it had made her day! Jessie looked very happy with herself, even as I brushed the crisp crumbs and salt from her snout. We carried on the visit – ashamed – and by the time we reached the second ward we were visiting everyone was asking if Jessie was still hungry. The parents thought it so hilarious they'd told everyone!

21

Study, study and more study!

NOT LONG AFTER I RETURNED TO THE UK, I dropped an email to Ann Howie and reintroduced myself, hoping that she would remember me from the conference. Ann is based in Washington State but she has contacts all over the States, which had me wondering if I could arrange something for when Mike was out in Seattle for three weeks in June 2016.

My mind was having a whirring moment and Ann provided the perfect resolution: the contact details for the person she knew who organised Seattle hospital's therapy dog team. Also, she invited me to spend a day with her, including a visit to Olympia Hospital, as long as I was prepared to drive the hour from Seattle to Olympia. Without hesitation I said yes ... and then booked a flight out to stay with Mike during the last week of his observership at the hospital. He would be busy during the day in theatre and clinic with a world-leading paediatric foot surgeon and I would be busy with my own AAI interests plus, of course, I still had coursework to do.

The dogs were easily sorted at home, once again enjoying being fussed over by Harry and Ollie, who had just finished their A-levels and GCSEs respectively, so were ready to enjoy some outdoor time and relax with their favourite companions, especially after being glued to their exam timetables for so long.

It was a dizzy time, but I was on a roll and the Seattle opportunity seemed too good to miss. It was lovely to see Mike but I knew that he had all of his days planned at the hospital, with long lists of operative procedures that he was to assist with, and I needed to make the best of my time out there. I headed off to the hospital, where a member of the volunteer team kindly took me on a tour of the facility and a walk of the wards. This was a revelation to me. I took a mental note of how they presented their therapy dog services on noticeboards using charts and photographs. Again, I wondered whether we could develop things at SCH to give more information about what we did so that people who had not heard about AAI were less surprised when they saw us heading down the corridors. Seattle Children's Hospital also had the most incredible roof terraces, where children were able to safely access the outdoors whenever they were well enough. I could see how much of a benefit that could be, too, and couldn't help thinking about Jo and the time we had met in the Macmillan Centre. There was a garden there too … perhaps we could use that in the future if an oncology patient wanted to see us outside in the fresh air? (Something we have since done on quite a few occasions.) I started to see that things with AAI didn't just have to be the same meet-and-greet model, always indoors and at the bedside.

The following day I drove to Olympia Hospital to see Ann, where she introduced me to a team at an adult rehabilitation unit that she ran and they gave me a demonstration of their canine AAI work. As ever, I had a million questions; all were answered or demonstrated patiently and with great detail by the team so I could work out what, if any of the services we could provide back home at an NHS hospital. As if that wasn't eye-boggling enough, Ann and I went for lunch and afterwards she took me to her training facility. Again there was more inspiration. There I could see how the dogs' training involved experiences they might encounter in a hospital environment way before they stepped into the real thing. As with everything with dog training, it was all about learning experiences and rewarding the positives so that when a dog saw a walking frame or a wheelchair, for example, it was not an issue. What I witnessed that day was Ann's expertise in canine body language as well as how to assess therapy dogs for particular roles in hospitals, what they and the handlers needed to know, and she had the skills to be able to pass on that knowledge to her teams.

I headed back to the hotel and completed some coursework on my laptop, with a pen and paper beside me so I could make notes all the time as everything that I had encountered came flooding back. I'm not sure that Mike got a word in edgeways over dinner. I just needed to share everything I had seen and heard and try to process it all in relation to working with my therapy dogs. He was really helpful, tired but happy to roll with my enthusiasm and fountain of ideas – workable and impossible. Mike is always an honest sounding board and he knows how hospitals work, so I trust his judgement implicitly. But in Seattle I'm sure he thought I had gone crazy as I presented all these marvellous seeds of ideas!

Week by week, the course ramped up. If I wasn't writing, I was reading and because I'm not someone who can read and read without falling asleep, I decided pretty quickly that the volume of reading was likely to sink me if I tried to do it all after I'd completed my routine roles, including work for my business, a dog visit and a couple of dog walks – not necessarily in that order. By the time I sat down to read there were times when my heavy eyelids felt as though they had glue on them. So, I read on our cross trainer. I had all the books on both Kindle as well as hardback, which meant I was able to study wherever I was and make notes on my Kindle if I was exercising. By the end of the course in November, I had leg muscles to die for and a head full of knowledge!

Some coursework was allied to what I had read and my field of AAI, while other modules were completely at odds. I remember feeling concerned when we did the animal ethics module and looked at the dogs lying at my feet as we watched videos which asked us to judge whether they were comfortable or not when doing different versions of AAI. I felt sure my dogs enjoyed what they did, but I started checking them more than I ever had once I was back in the hospital. I had already reduced the length of time we visited after taking Leo's breeder Catherine in on a specially permitted observation visit. She said she was very proud of the work we were doing but could identify on that occasion when Leo had 'run out of gas'. I was mortified but nevertheless incredibly grateful for her honesty.

I suddenly realised the danger of being too close to see exactly what is going on. But there was a reason I was guilty of asking so much of my dogs at that time: I had yet to learn the art and the sense of saying 'no'! The constant adding of just 'one more patient, please' always turned into more as it's so difficult to turn on your heels if the children opposite that 'one more child' are desperate to say hello and almost hanging out of their beds to stroke the dog. That 'yes' to just one more had to stop for everyone's benefit.

One of the pieces of learning that helped me with this decision-making was the canine body language module and it was something I could put into practice right away. I thought I was pretty good at reading the signs in my dogs but, once again, the course material was a revelation to me: I was picking up on the odd thing, but was I attuned to messages given out by their regular body language, including tiredness? When *they* needed attention rather than always giving attention? Was I getting it right all the time? The course gave me a great deal of thought on the ethics of what we were doing. As the handler, I was the dogs' advocate, in the same way as the parent was usually the child's advocate at the hospital. I had to be sure that the dogs were enjoying their role when I was asking them to partner me on a visit. Without that it was not going to work.

Anything that helped with my dog's health and wellbeing was of great interest to me. They didn't ask to be brought into this role, this bargain with myself that I must give back. That was my decision. The last thing I wanted for my dogs was any upset or distress. Nothing must cause them harm. They were my priority in this from day one and always would be.

Canine assisted intervention is what I am all about and I can't see me swapping to horses or donkeys any time soon, but it was fascinating to look at all the animal applications showing how all types of animals can be incorporated into AAI. As part of the course, I was granted permission to visit a donkey sanctuary for the day to see how children on the autism spectrum are supported by these gentle creatures and to see the children react to their solid, non-threatening presence. I saw how donkeys give themselves to the children in a dignified, friendly, stoic way that I had never appreciated before.

Some of the modules of my course had more to do with the other students but they *all* gave me some form of inspiration. At the time I wondered if I would ever use the Animal Assisted Education knowledge, but as time has passed, we have utilised it both in the school rooms and also at the bedside of some of the children. All it requires is a way of involving the animals. When I studied, I created a maths lesson for little ones. More recently during the Covid lockdown, some of the hospital school children have had a Zoom lesson about space which has involved our team of dogs led by our very own 'Dogstronaut Quinn Peake'. I am sure the SENCO (special education needs coordinator) teacher who asked us to devise something thought I was quite mad when I said we could do planets bingo with a team of dogs, but it was all great fun.

The one module I found the hardest to mentally compute was on the Colorado Link project. This saw us discuss the correlation between human versions of abuse and animal abuse, and most of the reading and discussions were tough going. The content was responsible for a few sleepless nights and at first, I wondered how this could impact on my work. Then I realised this was a lesson for me both in understanding some aspects of life that, thankfully, I have not been exposed to, and also in how to talk to children who may not necessarily have strong bonds with their own adults or those people around them in life. All these little nuggets of information that initially seemed superfluous to a volunteer walking the wards at a UK children's hospital have all proved very valuable in many ways since.

There were times during the year that I felt I was going to drown in textbooks, assignments and my own developing ideas on AAI and then a day visiting the children's wards with Leo put all that into perspective. When we heard that an intensive care doctor on the team treating three-year-old Oscar Haskell had asked for a visit from therapy dog Leo, we knew that it was an urgent request. Oscar was in PICU and ultimately was diagnosed as suffering from a rare brain condition called ADEM: he couldn't move, speak, react, and then his heart rate increased to a dangerous level. The family had given the go-ahead for Leo's visit and we were soon able to be at Oscar's bedside.

When we stepped into the bay, Leo typically reacted to the tense situation by radiating his calm to everyone around. He stood and waited for me to do what I do; the bed was lowered, the nurses had cleared an area of the tubes and I laid a mat over the bedding, as it was so important there was no contact with all the tubes going into Oscar's body. Then I placed Oscar's hand on Leo's paw. It was then that it happened – Oscar smiled! No one expected that. It was against all the odds as, up until then, his blank face had shown no sign of smiling at all. No one could have predicted that but it happened and his vital signs stabilised a little too. At that moment, a little bit of hope arrived!

It was a wonderful moment, even some of the clinical team said that it was incredible. Oscar's mum, Zoe, was in tears, calling it a miracle, and some of the intensive care team had to look away as they discreetly avoided showing a tear. Leo looked to me with an expression of understanding as if he was aware of what had happened and looked pretty pleased with himself. He certainly enjoyed all the fuss that came with it. He loves a friendly crowd and he certainly had an adoring audience that day. There it was, Animal Assisted Intervention in action, right before our eyes. I was on my way to finishing my course and there I was witnessing a perfect example of why I do what I do. Leo connected with Oscar and the smile appeared like a ray of sunshine. I could not have been more proud of my dog and neither could Oscar's parents or the hospital.

Later that year, just before Christmas, the media came knocking again and this time, having done lots more with Oscar once he had had left intensive care, AAI was hailed a true miracle by Oscar's parents, who spoke to *BBC Breakfast* television.

Shortly before that, in November I made another trip to Denver to present my capstone project, the final part of the course, which encompassed all that I had learned and how theoretically it could be put into my 'practice' in a perfect world. The strengths and weaknesses, what could be achieved and what would be desirable, together with considerations for other aspects of a service in line with what I had learned. One by one, having submitted the full written documents a few days earlier, all of our cohort presented the basis of our individual projects. I can't tell you how many times I went through that talk in the week before. When Mike rang to wish me good luck at 8am that morning I had been using the power of my jetlag – that woke me at 4am – to recite my presentation on a loop!

It felt brilliant to be standing there delivering the presentation that would, hopefully, bring me the qualification I had worked so hard for but never thought possible. It was a little bit like an out-of-body experience: there but watching myself, from above. I wanted this so much and I gave it so much of myself. It was such a relief when I spoke the final word and I could finally sit down. I could do no more. As soon as everyone had presented, we went outside and it was wonderful. By that time, I needed to breathe in some of the fresh Colorado air.

Lucky for me the course tutors had arranged another activity for all of us the following day. So, after spending some time on campus, we were treated to a trip to a large animal sanctuary at the foot of the Rockies, where AAI is offered to children and teens using a variety of animals including reptiles, birds, goats, sheep, cows, horses, cats, dogs and – would you believe it – camels! Inspired – and just a little less fearful of cows, horses and camels than flapping birds – I found it a great experience, one that really brought home to me that 'the connection' in the human-animal bond is the key to it all. I love my dogs and I see their brand of AAI working every day at home and in the hospital, but if someone else receives that connection with a horse, a cat or a camel, it really doesn't matter. If it happens, then it's real and it's honest because animals don't fake anything. I could see right there why I've always considered that the human-animal bond is worth its weight in gold.

I returned home with my course complete and my Certificate in Animal Assisted Therapy, Activities and Learning. I was exhausted, but happy! Turning 50 in January 2017 was a landmark that now has something worthwhile attached to it. I treated myself to the course and the flights as my advance birthday present to myself and I have no regrets. That gift has enriched me so much more than any other and I still count that year of study and enlightenment as one of my happiest years ever. Mike told me that he was so proud of me and remarked on what it said on the paperwork about having completed 350 contact hours: 'Blimey, no wonder you've been busy!' he said.

Going back into the hospital with my certificate behind me felt like a massive achievement. I had seen so much in Denver and learnt so much from the course and the other students that I simply had to make use of it at SCH. The big plus here was that I was no longer alone in this venture. With Monty in retirement I still had Totty, Jessie and Leo, and now Archie and Hattie on the canine team, and with fellow handlers Karen and Hannah beside me I knew that we could expand on what I'd started. And thanks to the media, the success with little Oscar was big news inside and outside the hospital. The question was ... What was I going to do first?

22

My world stops

SATURDAY, 30 DECEMBER 2017 was a fabulous day. The sun was out, the air crisp and cold, the ideal weather for a walk on the beach. Leo, as always, was not very keen on climbing into the car, much preferring to hang back with Monty, who had already had his 'joint kind' old man walk and was ready for a snooze at home. Once he realised that it was just to be him and the girls, he climbed in and we were soon off to Hill Head near Lee-on-Solent, our closest beach and one of our favourite haunts.

There was not much on the roads, so we made good time, parked and got ready to unload the dogs for their fun. It was as if this amazing day had been sent especially for us at the end of an incredibly busy year. To be able to breathe it all out into the sea air and breathe in the fresh stuff was pretty amazing and exactly what my head needed. Karen was there with dogs Hattie and Archie, who were eager to get onto the beach and play together with my three. As soon as the boot of the car was open, they all followed Karen down the boat ramp and onto the beach, dashing off to play down there on the long pebbly beach abandoned by a low jade tide. I looked on with pride. They looked magnificent tearing off at full speed towards the water. They were heading off to the shallows, where the wisps of sea foam blown in by the wind would tickle their paws. I followed them at my own pace with their leads, just in case I needed them, and as I did, I realised that I was one short. 'Damn ... trust me to do that!' I said, as I smiled to myself and turned back to the car.

Karen was already at the water's edge with the dogs sploshing and splashing around her, but then I spotted Leo heading towards me up the boat ramp, probably to check what I was up to. If any of the dogs was bound to do that, it was Leo. But this was time for him to have fun and let loose, so I shouted to him: 'Go on, Leo, go back ...!' He did just as I'd asked, but instead of going back the same way, for some reason he took a different route towards the seawall. I called to him and kept calling, but the wind must have taken my voice away (or perhaps he was ignoring me). Then, suddenly, he just disappeared from view. My heart stopped as I heard someone scream.

I ran down the boat ramp towards the direction I had seen him jump, calling Karen on her mobile to come over to where I was heading, and thank goodness she answered, but by then the other dogs had also noticed a commotion on the beach and were already on their way to me. Leo had jumped off the seawall but as it was low tide there was no sea for him to jump into. The sight that met me when we reached him sent shivers down my spine. He was curled up, his face planted into the shingle right beside a small child who just carried on collecting shells. He looked hurt and confused. In my best, quietly encouraging voice, I tried to get him to stand but he couldn't. His back was curved and he was bleeding from his mouth. My heart was racing.

Karen put the other dogs on leads while I spoke to the kind gentleman who offered help lifting Leo back to my car. Whoever that was, I want to thank him here I just didn't want to move my dog until I had spoken to Mike and explained what had happened.

Mike asked me how far Leo had fallen and we estimated it was an eleven- to twelve-foot drop from the seawall with no tide below it, so perhaps with a jump too he had fallen more than thirteen feet. Mike told me to be very careful lifting him, so I thanked those around me but insisted I should do it alone because if anything further happened to my boy it had to be my fault. Somehow, I carried him back to the car and called our vet Alex to say that I was bringing Leo right over.

My instinct was to drive as fast as legally possible, but it was vital that I drove steadily and carefully so that Leo wasn't swayed around in the back of the car. All the way home I felt like crying but I had to be strong. I thought of the worst-case scenario and at the same time hoped against hope that my brilliant boy was not permanently injured. What if he was? How would I tell the patients and staff? In that twenty-five-minute journey to Alex it all hit home again that Leo was not only my pet dog, he was an integral part of other people's lives too. I thought of the children in the hospital and those we had seen at the hospice who looked forward to his visits and spending time with him. If anything happened to Leo, how would I tell them? They would be heartbroken. I had a dawning realisation that along with the privilege of sharing Leo with the children came the responsibility of not wanting to let them down.

I popped home en route to drop Totty and Jessie off, and Ollie came out to see Leo. Poor Ollie, he looked ashen when he saw our friend lying there injured. Seconds later, we were on the way to Alex and it was such a relief to see her standing outside to meet us. She examined Leo in the back of the car, getting in with him first to check he was safe to move. There didn't seem to be any major damage in the form of broken bones. She checked his mouth and discovered that he had bitten his tongue and his chin had a split that looked quite deep. Alex squeezed it to determine just how deep and out popped a small shell. I couldn't help but laugh. I put it down to the shock.

Alex suggested that Leo must rest at home for twenty-four hours to see how things progressed with strict rest and pain relief. The blood from his tongue looked dramatic but the injury was self-healing and his chin didn't need stitches. In the couple of hours since 'taking flight' and completion of her assessments the hump on his back had relaxed a little and thankfully this was just put down to spasm. Leo was already up and trying to move but he had a worrying limp. So, we agreed that I would take him home and review later over the phone and the next day. I spent the night in the lounge with Leo, talking to him and willing him to be better the next time he tried to stand. I felt sick with worry as I held him close.

The following morning, he really could not put his right front paw down and needed my support to go outside for a quick pee. He winced with pain with every step so I carried him back into the house and checked in with Alex. I laughed at the fact that I was worried about Leo's back while probably doing mine an injury lifting him so much, but it was what I needed to do. Mike was at work again so couldn't help with hauling this 34kg patient of mine. It was New Year's Eve and we just had to wait until first thing on New Year's Day before the full inflammatory effect would show on Leo's joints. All the swelling after an injury takes forty-eight hours to come up so we just had to be patient. I am absolutely no good at waiting. With every hour I could see in his eyes that it was hurting him when he tried to move, but I had to follow Alex's advice to give it time and I trusted her totally. I just wished that I could rewind time and not go to the beach, not have yesterday at all, then Leo would be OK.

I said to myself: 'I'm going to lose *my* Leo.' Somehow I felt it and it made me think of some of the patients who'd had life-changing injuries. That thought kept going round in my head. When I shared my fears with Mike or the boys, they could not offer any genuinely reassuring words because no one knew how this was going to end. We all knew things didn't look great. I couldn't think about anything else – only Leo.

New Year's Day dawned and Leo was no better so, as arranged, Mike spoke to Alex about a referral. It was a no-brainer. Mike knew Leo needed to be seen by neuro-orthopaedic veterinary surgeon Professor Noel Fitzpatrick, so the referral was written, the call made and off I went to meet Noel at the practice later that day. For Noel to make the time to see us on New Year's Day was, I think, an exceptional act of kindness that Mike and I will never forget. Not having to wait that extra day made such a difference.

As I mentioned earlier, Leo and I had met Noel some years before when filming for his *Supervet in the Field* series for Channel 4. On the programme, Leo was reunited with one of his first SCH patients, Becky, whose leg was saved after Leo licked her toes. Since then, Mike had collaborated with Noel as a Trustee of the Humanimal Trust, but this was seeing the Supervet in his professional capacity, a situation I had hoped we would never need.

We were in Noel's consulting room with the dog skeleton on the counter, a scene very familiar to anyone who watches the *Supervet* series. But this was me ... with Leo. The X-rays and scans were done. While in the consulting room, like every worried dog mum, I probably listened to a fraction of what I was being told as I only wanted to hear that Leo was OK. I listened intently when Noel called Mike to discuss the treatment options. All the orthopaedic terms flew between the two of them rapidly and I tried to keep up, but of course I couldn't, so I just stroked Leo instead, hoping that he didn't blame me for what happened and what he was going through.

When the call ended, Noel turned to me and said: 'We'll give it a go. Mike and I have agreed that we will keep surgery in reserve and try rehab, but there is only one chance on this, Lyndsey. He has to really have you *and* luck on his side to get away with intensive physiotherapy to recover from this. It's a nasty injury.'

Noel reassured me that, thankfully, there was no spinal injury, despite first appearances. I'd certainly thought Leo's spine was broken when I'd first seen the curve of his back. The reason he was still limping was that he had ruptured the ligaments in his front paw, the equivalent joint to the human wrist. It is quite possible that Leo had dislocated the wrist in the fall, ruptured the ligaments but that luckily, the joint had relocated by itself. One option for treatment was immediate surgery to fix the wrist 'solidly', an operation called a fusion, which meant Leo would never move that joint again, although we could expect him to walk and run without pain once it had healed. The other was the physiotherapy and that was the path we set out on. I reassured Noel that he would never have met a more compliant owner and that the seventy-five-minute distance between home and the practice was not an issue. If he wanted us there three times a week, we would be there. And we were.

I was already well-acquainted with the frustrations that all orthopaedic surgeons have with patients who swear blind that they will work hard on their rehab to maximise their gains but then lose momentum after a few weeks, or maybe only days. I regularly hear Mike moaning about how some of the children he has operated on could have done better had they been more compliant with physiotherapy. I was going to do everything that Noel and his team advised me to do for Leo. It was my turn to do something for him and I was not going to let him down.

Leo was booked for his first session the following day. I carried him in using the hoist we had been told that he needed to wear in order to keep the weight out of his paw. Poor Leo, he looked like some kind of giant puppet on strings and my daft dog thought he was there to make everyone smile! Despite being the injured party, he was soon imploring one of the receptionists to give him a cuddle. And so, it started; Leo seemed to think he was now visiting Fitzpatrick Referrals not only for them to look at the tendons on his paw but also to carry out some sort of a therapy dog visit!

Intensive ultrasound and laser treatment followed by massage that I could continue at home that evening, and again on the days in between, gradually saw things change little by little. I knew that we had Leo in the best of professional hands, but at home it was all down to me to get this right and follow Noel and his team's guidance to the letter. The early days were easier than those that followed. Right after the accident, he didn't try to do anything much but as time went on, I needed to oversee what Leo was up to all the time to stop him doing too much. It was like having a young child that you had to think for all the time. When did he last pee? Must be due now, so put the hoist on, take him outside to have a pee, bring back in, etc. He couldn't wander off through the dog flap and do his thing, so it was a real test of my body language skills.

I realised that by then, we were actually in week two of rehab. That may sound odd but had we taken the surgical route we would have been six weeks behind this point as the wounds needed to heal before full rehab could start. This was the one chance I had to avoid surgery and with Noel directing his specialist physiotherapists we were giving Leo the very best chance. Mike and I had every faith in the team and I was determined not to fail.

It was the worst of times and I felt as if I couldn't close my eyes for a second. I didn't sleep or eat much at all, afraid that I would miss something vital that I needed to report back. I knew my patient well. Stoic Leo was not going to be one of those patients who complained all the time and commanded the attention reserved for others. Oh no, Leo was the patient who slept, nuzzled, demanded nothing of me other than what he was offered. That's why I had to keep a special eye on him.

Of course, I still had Monty and co to look after too but somehow, the dogs all knew that we wouldn't be heading out of the door first thing and abandoning our patient. They soon adapted to the new routine of waiting for their walks until someone else in the household was up and able to watch Leo.

At the same time, I still desperately wanted to visit the hospital. I felt forced to declare Leo's accident on our social media so people knew that he had been injured and I put a little video of him on Facebook to show him trying to walk. I hoped that would explain exactly why it was impossible for Leo to walk the long corridors of the hospital, but I didn't think it was a good enough excuse for me to take a leave of absence. I wasn't the one off my feet! So, I took Jessie to the hospital whenever I could and of course so many good wishes were passed to us to give to Leo while I was there and via our social media. The children on some of the wards even created huge cards for him and sent them by post!

Although I felt a huge pull to be back on the wards, I was reassured that things were well covered by the rest of the team. Karen and Hannah went in as much as they could with Archie and Hattie. Somehow between us we were still seeing patients and I am pretty sure we didn't let anyone down. Nevertheless, as the days turned into weeks, then a month, I still worried whether Leo would ever return.

I was torn between two worlds: where I needed to be for Leo and where I felt I needed to be for the patients. The dilemma had me in a mental vice and the only way I could free myself from it was to try and do both things to the best of my ability – to KBO – keep battling on! As I walked the corridors of the hospital with Jessie, I told her that we were doing our best for Leo and that when he was back on the team everything would be right in our world – she would see that. No need to worry. Everything was going to be fine. I needed to remember that Jessie probably knew that without my reassurances. She was doing a great job but then she has a real talent for making people smile. Thinking about that now, I remember one evening when Mike was working late and I still had children to see with Jessie, who was 'appearing' as her alter ego, 'the hairy fairy'.

I appreciate and respect that many people in the world of AAI believe that we must not anthropomorphise animals and that perhaps it somehow degrades them, especially if we dress them in 'human' clothes. I can see their point if we dressed them all the time, but they are only in a costume briefly, one which has been specifically created or adapted. When you are working with children, if the dogs are happy and not restricted, irritated or overheated then a pair of fairy wings attached to a proper canine harness on an extrovert golden retriever is only a recipe for smiles.

That particular evening, while Jessie took her applause for prancing around, looking adorable and cheering everyone up, Mike was finishing his theatre list. The porters took the final patient into the theatre suite and the talk is that there is a dog on the wards making everyone smile. Mike knows I am there. He performs the final operation of the day and sends me a text to see if I am still around and, fortunately, he just catches me as we're heading out of the door. He says that the theatre team are really keen to see what they always hear about but miss seeing for themselves. With that, I nipped back in and upstairs, hurriedly put the wings back on the dog and, ready to meet everyone outside the theatre suite, Jessie the hairy fairy is met by more smiling faces keen to have a team photo session. It's all smiles at the end of hours in the operating theatre, thanks to a dog in her fairy wings, happy to see everyone and share the love.

As we finally head out of the hospital buoyed by our visit and Jessie's star performance, I think of Leo and how he loves being with me, doing what we do, and in my mind's eye, I can see him in his Harry Potter spectacles, giving very scared and poorly children something to smile about. I want to see him back there, where he belongs.

23

Come on, Leo ...

WE HAD BEEN GOING TO FITZPATRICK REFERRALS for a while when one of our appointments fell on Valentine's Day, so we took some gifts for the team who had now become Leo's best friends. On his previous visit he had wowed them in his lion's mane wig and received all the attention and smiles to which he was accustomed as a therapy dog on his hospital rounds. I realised that, for him, despite the fact that he was the patient not the visitor, going for physio was his only proper outing and somehow, I think, it was keeping him psychologically chipper. He seemed to thrive on the fact that just the two of us spent three and a half hours together travelling somewhere where patients were treated and then we came home. I wonder if he thought he was going there to do AAI in some way. I can't be sure but I can tell you that his happiest days of the whole recovery cycle were the days spent travelling to Noel's practice, and I was happy as long as we were making progress.

One day, when we had been going there for about eight weeks, Noel came to chat to me about Leo's progress. His physio had reported that his recovery had plateaued. I must have looked panicked as I asked if that now meant surgery, but inside my head I wondered if it was another way of saying that all my efforts had failed. Before my insecurity ran away with me, Noel confirmed that it did look as though Leo had plateaued but he had come a long way and that I had done all that was asked of me, all that I could.

'Don't worry, we can try something,' Noel continued. 'If you can hang around a bit, we can give him some sedation and try some shockwave. He can only have three sessions of that but it's worth a try.' I knew that there was an explanation that went with that but it was wasted on me. 'OK, Noel, that means nothing to me but what did Mike think of the idea?' He said that he would chat to him and cue more 'orthobabble': words like 'outcome', 'efficacy', 'stats, 'protocol', 'research' ... all these words bouncing down the phone line. All I knew was that I had to text my friend Carole, who had the other dogs at home, to say that I would be away so much longer than planned.

I left Leo in the capable hands of Noel and his team and headed into Guildford. I needed to leave but as I drove away, I felt my anxiety return with a body blow. Where was I going? Silly woman! Why hadn't I stayed there and sat in the waiting room? It made me think of the hospital and how some of the parents are just so desperate to leave the building to take in some fresh air when anxiety hits and here I was heading to Sainsbury's in Guildford. Sainsbury's for no other reason than a mooch around and to waste time.

I believe that, whether it is your child or your beloved pet, when a surgeon takes them into an area where you cannot follow, you just need to do whatever suits you. I wanted to take Leo's injury away. I wanted him back to normal, as if this had never happened and we were really only at the vet's for a check-up and then heading off for a walk in the country park or at the beach. NO! Would I ever want to go to the beach again? I didn't know if I could answer that yet. I left Sainsbury's with things I didn't need and returned to the practice to wait.

I was called into one of the consulting rooms and in came a very dopey-looking Leo with one of the veterinary nurses and Noel. 'Come on, buddy,' he said to Leo, who looked as if he needed a long sleep. 'Easy does it, but let's show your ma what we've done.' Noel went on to show me the range of movement that Leo could now do with his right paw and told me that I should continue to massage and stretch this but also continue being very careful. The idea was that if this worked, it would expedite the healing of the damaged ligament and joint capsule, and within the next couple of weeks of physio, we would see another phase of progress. After those two to three weeks, if he plateaued again, he could have another session ... which is what happened.

We continued with the massage and gentle stretching as the specialist physio had taught me and I felt as though I was doing it non-stop, or so it seemed at the time! Every time I had finished walking the others, doing something at home, been on a hospital visit or done some work for my business, I realised about four more hours had passed and

I should again do it for just a few minutes to help Leo's paw. Had it become an obsession? Yes, of course it had, but we had come this far and I wasn't going to stop now. On that second appointment, a few weeks later, I stayed in the reception area, reading. My mind was much more at ease because I was where I needed to be.

After four months of treatment, involving shockwave and intensive specialist physiotherapy with ultrasound and laser, Leo was back to running around and, best news of all, Noel was able to give him the all-clear to return to work. I was elated! After our follow-up visit, Noel wrote to Mike to give the final clinical details and he mentioned how compliant an owner I had been. I was pleased with that and when he went on to say he was quite sure at the beginning that without my dedication to the cause, Leo would have needed surgery, I realised how close we had come to having no choice in the matter. We could not thank Noel enough for what can only be described as his supreme expertise and professionalism. It was thanks to his guidance and the dedication of his team to healing Leo's paw that success was achieved without surgery. Mike wrote back to Noel to thank him and said something to the effect of: '... Lyndsey's commitment to our canine family cannot be underestimated.' That was good to hear too, but it wasn't the praise or the cost that mattered to me – I had my boy back!

Leo had accepted his treatment with the same patience and dignity as many of the young patients he visits. Everyone he met at Fitzpatrick's agreed that he is one special dog. I gauged that it was time for Leo to gradually resume his hospital-visiting duties at SCH. It was set to be an emotional return for a dog who was so loved by everyone – patients, staff and parents alike.

During the four months Leo had been in recovery, we'd been inundated with 'Get Well, Leo' cards and messages. The children drew pictures for him and some of his regular patients, the long stayers for whom his visit was the highlight of their week, wrote some heart-rending messages. It was overwhelming but in a very good way. It left me in no doubt at all that Leo was not only precious to me, but he was also precious to many others. I made the choice to share my lovely dog with others, to take him to them, so I've no idea why I was so surprised at the deep love and concern that others openly showed for him. I was the lucky one. I had the pleasure of seeing others benefit from his company but I was the one who took him home at night. My belief in Leo as a therapy dog was total and I wanted him to feel that same belief in me when he needed it most.

Leo, my 'partner in care', hospital hero and it seemed, everyone's dog in a million.

It was ironic that Leo's terrible accident came at the end of a year filled with incredible steps forward for the therapy dog team in terms of AAI and recognition for what we were achieving at Southampton Children's Hospital. While I watched over Leo as he made his recovery, I thought about the hurdles that we had cleared and the advances that put the trips to Denver and the completion of my Certificate in Animal Assisted Therapy,

Activities and Learning into perspective. It was all starting to make sense and the pieces of the SCH AAI jigsaw were falling into place.

24

Nurses believing in AAI – worth its weight in gold

> 'She was alone, in an unfamiliar ward, having just woken up from a huge surgery and an anaesthetic; she wasn't used to dogs and we were all strangers, but somehow the presence of Leo made it work ...'
>
> Donna Austin: Advanced Nurse Practitioner in Paediatric Intensive Care, SCH

I remember this case and the vulnerability of that young girl. And I remember Leo approaching her as usual, calmly offering himself to reassure her. He was there for her in that moment and she accepted him. I also remember that the nurse attending this patient was not one that was especially keen on dogs being on the ward, but in Leo, that day, she saw something she never expected – a dog as a bridge to communicate with a lonely, anxious child. They had tried everything else and it took a dog to break the silence and the barriers and create trust. Leo, with his 'you're safe with me' eyes, made a connection that said, 'You are not alone, you can trust these people. Like me, they want to help you.'

Dogs 'do' trust very well. And if we trust in them, I believe that we are usually rewarded.

Sometimes people, nurses too, just have to see it for themselves.

The results of a survey conducted by the Royal College of Nursing (RCN) in 2016 revealed that half of the UK's nurses had, at some point in their career, encountered work with therapy animals and 98 per cent of them had seen it benefit their patients. The not-so-positive finding was that a quarter of those who took part in the survey were in a workplace that did not allow animals through the door. When Amanda Cheesley, Professional Lead for Long Term Conditions and End of Life Care at the Royal College of Nursing, said that she had heard about the work we were doing at SCH and wanted to come and have a look for herself with a crew from *BBC Breakfast*, I thought, bring it on – brilliant! This was our opportunity to showcase what we do to the wider nursing profession and the public who would see the programme.

They were able to see Leo in action with some of his long-term patients and performing a little Animal Assisted Activity in a meet-and-greet session which included an interview with Alice on how she felt our support had helped her through years of cancer treatment. She said stroking Leo was lovely because it 'reminded her of being at home.' The film also showed little Oscar doing some paw-print painting with Leo, which of course made him smile, just as he smiled for the first time looking at Leo.

After meeting the team, including the dogs, and enjoying

a tour of the children's wards, Amanda acknowledged that we were doing something more involved than most volunteer therapy dog teams that she knew of, beyond what she had encountered before. I took this as a huge compliment. I was delighted that she had invited us to take part and it really is a lovely piece to re-watch and listen to the parents of patients talking about the difference the dogs have made, not just to their child but the whole family.

From my learning and all those hours of study I realised that we had already been carrying out Animal Assisted Intervention before I knew it had a name. I just hadn't realised until I did all the reading and studied on the course, which revealed the field was so well defined already. We had been receiving referrals from the clinical teams to participate in the care and recovery of specific patients for a couple of years before I studied for the certificate. Our general meet-and-greet work, I realised, was Animal Assisted Activity, and Animal Assisted Education when we supported children during learning activities in the ward school room or at their bedside. When we partnered a healthcare professional to do some work based on a goal they were trying to achieve with a patient, and that was ultimately documented, then what we were doing was called Animal Assisted Therapy.

After gaining the certificate, I felt equipped to be more inventive and ultimately do much more with the knowledge and confidence I had gleaned from taking the plunge to study this fascinating subject. Maybe that's why Amanda asked me to join a new committee set up by the RCN to create the first set of guidelines to form a protocol for working with dogs in healthcare settings, to ensure best practice. I accepted the invitation immediately and clicked my mind into all the work I had already done on these topics.

To have the RCN interested in what we were up to was very exciting because it is generally the nursing staff we work with every time we visit and with whom we have, next to their patients, the closest relationship. To have healthcare professionals believe in the power of AAI is worth its weight in gold: it gives credibility to our presence on the ward and makes accessing us far easier. I didn't know at that stage what being on the committee would mean, other than being busier still, but I knew for certain that having a framework to work to and provide guidelines had to be good as protection for everyone involved in Animal Assisted Intervention, from the animal to the patient.

As news of the development of the guidelines became apparent, Amanda warned me that there was a possibility that more TV filming requests would come my way, especially as the committee worked towards the launch of the guidelines. I'm not sure that Karen and Hannah had ever imagined that volunteering to take their dogs to visit hospital patients would result in appearing on TV, but as part of the team they got caught up in the filming too – even if they preferred to leave all the talking to me!

The impact of what the dogs were achieving was being recognised within the hospital too:

> 'Morning, I have a five-year-old who I've been working with for a while, who is due surgery soon, and I'd like to do some work with an anaesthetic mask and visit the anaesthetic room. The anaesthetist has agreed, she should be around on the 15th, are you, guys?'

I received this request from our play specialist colleague, Jo, and I remember thinking it might be something we could help with but wouldn't it be great if I could train Leo to wear the same mask that the little girl Lillian feared? The next time I was in the hospital I asked for the type of anaesthetic mask that might be used – a large one that would fit a retriever muzzle. Over the next couple of weeks, I gently introduced the mask to Leo, with a little help from some peanut butter smeared inside! No wonder it wasn't long before his big hairy snout was in the mask ... and no surprise that the other dogs wanted a turn too. The power of peanut butter never fails. We were ready to give it a go with our patient.

When we met Lillian she only had a few weeks to go before her operation, so catching her at her pre-op consultation was good timing. Leo was very gentle with Lillian, offering himself for her to stroke as we played and chatted, and I showed her pictures of the dogs and gave her stickers – all the usual things. Jo had her pre-operative toy box on hand with toys that encourage chat about being in hospital and she broached the subject of the operation. This was our chance to introduce the idea that Leo might be able to be there to help make things easier for her if she could tell him what she was worried about. Lillian looked a bit puzzled about that, but with a bit of a prompt from Jo, the little one went on to explain about the mask and how she was afraid of it. Then it was my turn: I asked Lillian if she would 'teach' Leo and me to wear a mask.

Without any more prompts Lillian took great delight in teaching first me and then Leo how to wear the mask. By the end of our lesson, she was sitting on my knee, playfully wearing the once-dreaded mask, with me and Leo wearing ours too! Job done, photo taken and a memory created. Lillian had no idea that Leo had already been trained at home in the weeks prior to our meeting and it was not his first mask encounter, but that was fine. As far as our patient was concerned, she had helped me teach him. But how could we make sure that we could replicate it a few weeks later on the day of the op?

I suggested to Lillian's mum that I message her with a picture of Leo practising with his mask at home every couple of days leading up to the day of the operation. And that's exactly what we did, with Lillian knowing that Leo would be with her on her big day, too.

When we arrived, Lillian had been admitted to the ward and was already in her surgical gown and sitting comfortably on her bed doing some colouring to pass the time. We chatted, played some guessing games and spent time with her and her mum while we waited for the team to get everything ready. Then, when the time came for her to have her 'magic' numbing cream on the back of her hand, Leo mirrored that by having a canine-friendly cream smeared on the back of his paw, which was then wrapped up just like Lillian's hand. When the porters arrived, Leo and I escorted her on her trolley to the anaesthetic room. From the trolley, Lillian held Leo's second lead as alongside her mum, we walked down the corridor into the lift and ultimately to the theatre suite reception. It was difficult to watch this little girl who at such a young age was coping with a fear of an anaesthetic mask, most likely due to the number of operations she had already undergone. It still wasn't easy but Lillian's mum said that Leo had certainly helped her daughter face her fear.

I was feeling very proud of my dogs doing their own special brand of hospital work. At home there was every reason for me to feel proud of Jessie, who gave birth to her final litter of pups in February 2017. I decided to keep little Quinn, who was and still is so adorable. His name was special to us because it celebrated that we now had five dogs – our own canine quintet! The pups' arrival was exactly what one of our patients, Alice Razza, had been waiting for. I introduced you to Alice earlier, she was one of our first patients on the children's cancer ward. She had suffered a relapse and through her chemo and radical surgery, the dogs had been there to comfort her at every stage. As we had known her for so long, Alice had met all the dogs, the first being Monty way back when she found the courage to come from her room to see him not long after we accepted that initial invitation to visit the wards in 2013.

At other times in her hospitalisation, when she was having difficulty walking, Alice was reluctant to try taking any steps until Karen and Archie came to the rescue: she went for a walk and managed to do the stairs holding on to him, much to the delight and relief of her physiotherapist. And when she had radiotherapy, Leo accompanied her to the session to take away some of her anxiety over a new form of treatment when she was already so poorly.

When Alice was told that she was not responding to treatment and her path was going to be palliative, she decided that all she wanted to do was see the dogs. In the later days, when her energy was low, spending time with Jessie and the pups became the focus of her days, playing with them at my home and cuddling them as she watched them grow. And when life got really tough for Alice and she could no longer travel, I took Leo and little Quinn to see her at home. It was tough to watch. Monty, Totty, Jessie, Leo, Archie, Hattie and even puppy Quinn had all supported Alice on her cancer journey to the end.

Alice died in May 2017; she was 15 years old with still so much life to live and so many things to do. Her family carry with them so many memories of their daughter with the dogs who were there for her in her final days. The dogs couldn't heal her pain but they did what they always have the capacity to do – distract and soothe in a way that only they can. For Alice, the dogs were a life on which to attach a dream, to attach hope. It's why her mum and dad wanted to be beside us for our special day at *Crufts* in 2020.

It's all to do with the dogs, the invisible bond of empathy, trust and love that is forged with a child and secures some special memories for everyone – a love that has no end.

25

The priceless bond

HOSPITALS CAN BE SCARY, alien environments and working on the AAI section of the new Royal College of Nursing protocol was forcing me to look at what we were doing at SCH and strip that back to basics. It was pretty much a box-ticking exercise because I already knew that we were doing everything to satisfy the infection control team – the dogs were head-to-paw clean and we constantly reviewed their temperament and demeanour to make sure they were happy in their role. I often felt fortunate to have plenty of dogs to choose from. If there was ever a concern that one appeared tired or potentially unwell, I simply prepared one of my others as they were all on the team. The handlers had completed their volunteer protocols at the hospital, we had done our safeguarding modules and all of us had an empathic approach to the patients and knew how to work with our dogs. I knew all of this and I was happy with everything, but somewhere in my head I felt that, because I was contributing to these RCN guidelines, my own house had better be in bloody good order.

I heaped that pressure on all by myself, which was stupid as things were busy enough. As interest in the developing RCN guidelines started to take off, Amanda decided we should do a public lecture at the RCN. I wondered how on earth I would cope with doing that but, as ever, with my Leo by my side I decided that I could manage it and set about compiling a PowerPoint presentation.

It was OK. I knew that I could handle this; after all, I had survived delivering my final presentation for my studies in the States so, as long as I had the right information to deliver to the audience, I was home and dry. But, me being me, I couldn't leave it at that. I had another idea: I contacted Becky, who had appeared with Leo and I on the *Supervet* episode, and told her that I had a cunning plan if she was happy to be part of it. By then she was a nursing student in London. I just wondered if she was OK with me telling her story at the lecture and, thinking about it, would she like to be there in person? And one final question: if she was there, how would she feel if I pulled her out of the audience? All of that was met with a resounding: 'Yes, yes, yes!' So that was it, fixed. I would now not suffer a potential death by PowerPoint – thanks to Becky! She was my secret weapon, alongside Leo.

I kept her story to the end, when I told everyone the story of the girl in the pictures in the presentation, how we first met and about her treatment. I looked at Leo sitting with Mike in the audience for a shot of calm as I explained the importance of how Leo's intervention helped Becky and how she not only survived mental torment, a near-fatal fall and a long and painful recovery, she was now thriving and doing something truly amazing in training to be a nurse. And then I introduced her and asked her to stand. Thinking of that moment and how well she was received still gives me goosebumps. (She is now a registered nurse who has been working in London and is soon to start in cardiac intensive care at Great Ormond Street Hospital.)

That event was a massive step for me and although I was feeling the pressure of the task in hand, I had proved something to myself – I was no longer afraid of my own shadow or the dark clouds of doom that liked to gather whenever I felt vulnerable. I didn't feel alone or misplaced because I had Leo and Mike there and I was seeing the development of my AAI dream come to life in ways I'd never envisaged. I was presenting at the Royal College of Nursing, no less. Once again, I was seeing myself in a kind of out-of-body experience and, for the first time in a long while, I recognised the confident woman I was looking at – that woman was me.

The challenges of that year seemed to be coming thick and fast. When we gained a new voluntary services manager, she suggested we return to visiting patients of all ages – so going back on the previous manager's request to concentrate on children. I had to resist this because we had been working with the children at SCH for almost five years and had developed a great relationship with the staff to the point that we were getting more direct AAI referrals, like Annie who came to us from a consultant anaesthetist asking if Leo could help calm his patient before her surgery. She required extra support, having had an unsuccessful operation necessitating an emergency admission to PICU on a previous occasion. Annie was so anxious about having another operation but we knew that she loved dogs and her mum was willing to give it a go. On the day of the operation I had already gained permission for Leo to lie by Annie's side on some protective sheeting so he could support his patient for her pre-op tests, the chat with her consultant and her pre-med. In his own snoozy way, as the pre-med started to work on Annie, Leo enjoyed a big cuddle and soon both were looking very sleepy! Success for Annie was seeing her trust in Leo at a very anxious time in her young life.

What we were doing was really working. More than that, the dogs and handlers on the team were really suited to working with children. It was all going so well, so it seemed ironic that while I was working with the RCN on the protocol to guide the service, we were being asked to contemplate changes to how we worked.

It was a tricky and frustrating situation because the therapy dogs were, by then, an integral part of SCH. We were considered part of the Youth and Play Service team, who were responsible for many of our referrals. To get this far, we had already encountered some of the issues that had started to resurface, such as which handlers and dogs should visit the children's wards. The staff at SCH had built their trust not only in our dogs but in us as handlers and had seen benefits, some of which include: having a team made up of the same breed of dog works because we can rotate the dogs and handlers and the children can't manipulate anyone by saying they will only do something for a particular type of dog. It also means we don't risk attachment, which is not good for the patient or the team. And alongside all of that, we had a great system in place: the children collect their cards, stickers and see them as mascots for their hospitalisation. We were also documenting all of our visits, so building a huge amount of data on what we were doing. I didn't want to give that up or compromise it. As leader of the pack, or should I say lead therapy dog handler, I had to keep working to make our role better, not dilute it. Thankfully, after a few discussions it was resolved: we should continue developing what had become so successful and full support be given to our AAI team.

Sometimes I have to remind myself that I am a volunteer, not paid staff, but then this is the role that I chose to take and study for and all I want to ever do is to get it right for the dogs and the patients. Karen calls visiting with Archie her 'happy place', for me it has turned into a life passion – with dogs attached.

'I want to buy your dog!' I wasn't sure I had heard the guy correctly. So, he gave me a second chance: 'How much for your dog?' I'd been with Leo in the paediatric cardiac ward with a patient from overseas, whose parents spoke very little English. I'd seen the little girl lying in the side bay and thought about going in – the staff said I could but doubted I would get a response as she looked so sleepy when I peeped through the porthole window in the door on Ocean ward. As always, it had to be worth a try and anyway, the parents beckoned me into the room, where there was another man sitting in the corner of the room on his phone. He barely looked up, which made me feel a bit uneasy and

I wondered if he was working on his phone or perhaps just didn't like dogs (or me!). It was lovely to see the child smile as Leo engaged his usual charm offensive in his lovely placid way, but still she didn't speak. The card and stickers got him another smile but as I turned to leave, the girl spoke to her father. There was a brief exchange between the two men, who kept glancing at Leo. It all felt a bit unusual and I didn't understand a word that was being said, so I left and quickly reported in to the nursing station that all had gone well and that we were finished, and left the ward.

The man in the corner followed me out. 'Ah, Miss, I need to talk to you,' he said. 'The family want to buy the dog.' I wondered if I'd heard him right.

'Er, the dog is not for sale. He's my dog.' For some reason I felt angry. To think that's possible – to buy someone's beloved pet from them just like that. But somehow I kept my work face in place and remained calm and polite.

'Ma'am, you don't understand, I can offer you whatever you want, you name the price!'

I still laugh when I think about this story because it makes me realise how much of a massive misunderstanding there is about the real value of a dog – and it's not money. The value of Leo's presence in my life is priceless, as with all of my dogs. They are so interwoven into the fabric of my life that I would not part with any of them and they could not be pulled away from me by anyone, in any direction, whatever the price. When I'd first seen Leo after his leap over the seawall, I thought I would lose him and a crumb of that feeling has never left me.

26

Leo ... friend and soulmate

I WILL ALWAYS REMEMBER 2018, not just because the first part of the year – days, nights and inside my head – was dominated by Leo's recovery but also because my AAI dream was, scarily, becoming a reality. Truth is, I wasn't sure that I could handle everything going on all at the same time.

I felt overwhelm hovering over my shoulder again and my old enemy, self-doubt, limbering up for a good laugh at my expense. But then I looked at Leo – solid, majestic, handsome and caring Leo – and no one, but no one, was going to let him down. His innate qualities and unique dog patience were a big part of all that we had achieved so far, especially with children. He is a natural therapy dog: calm, patient, present, respectful and kind. As his handler, I learned a lot from him and added my learning and my determination to take the service to the SCH patients who needed us. We were in this together – for the long haul.

Leo didn't seem to have any physical after-effects following his crash-landing on the beach, but we will always have to be careful that he doesn't overdo the retrieval games he loves otherwise a limp returns. But it's really hard to limit him because Leo will run and retrieve for as long as you throw a ball or gundog dummy for him, and then when you stop, he gives you his best 'sad dog' eyes, which seem to say: 'But I'm only bringing you a present.' In one game, when he refused to let go of his new squeaky ball, I went up to him and noticed that one of his front teeth was missing! It had definitely been there a few days earlier when I gave all the dogs a dental check, so we suspect that he fractured the tooth when he fell and the ball had finally knocked it out. Leo's first post-accident visit to the beach was, mercifully, uneventful, but after Quinn cut his foot close to the dreaded accident point, we decided to avoid that part of the beach altogether.

It was great to have Leo beside me again, plodding along the hospital corridors with a big smile on his face and occasionally back in his 'dress-up' mode, which he adores, probably because he gets so much attention. Seeing Leo back in his lion's mane wig made the children giggle and want to play with him, sit with him and get as close as they could. And he loved it! The 'lion's mane' is just a silly thing that I saw online and ordered from America, although had I realised the import duty would be so much, I'd probably not have bothered! But for once, it paid off that ignorance was bliss because the wig has generated so many good memories and wonderful moments captured on the cameras of so many parents that those golden locks have paid me back a million times over in happiness.

Even the teenagers found the lion's mane humorous. Katie Scannell, sadly now one of our angel patients, was one who loved to see Leo in his lion's mane. Her all-time favourite was Archie really, but she called him and Leo 'her boys' right through her treatment, and ultimately 'her boys' were there when her family and friends said goodbye at her funeral. If the lion's mane causes people to double-take, I could say the same of the Harry Potter spectacles, the Pudsey outfit and Santa's helper, to name but a few. And that's not just Leo dressing up – the girls do the hairy fairy! It was lovely to have a line-up of Leo, Hattie and Milo celebrating World Book day at SCH, minus Archie who usually gives dress-up a miss. He prefers to suppress his family's theatrical gene and do his own thing, although he did once enjoy the Harry Potter outfit and glasses, so perhaps he is only willing to be a wizard.

Having said that, Leo, who is happy to be put 'in character', was very unhappy when a giant Peppa Pig paid a visit to SCH. Let's just say, they didn't hit it off! Poor Leo really did look terrified when he saw the six-foot pink pig heading down the corridor towards him. Things didn't go so well either with the BBC's canine puppet, Dodge. Poor Leo couldn't understand why sniffing Dodge's bottom was so unlike checking out any other dog. It really confused him! Nevertheless, he loved all the fuss the day that he joined Archie to pick up their CBeebies 'Hospital Heroes' award with patients Georgia and Gracie who'd nominated them.

Seeing Leo back on meet-and-greet duty and then getting into his extended AAI role with a patient was magical. It was pure Leo in action. It was as if he had never been away and meant I could push away memories of the awful day of his accident.

All the children we see are special and illness can make them vulnerable and scared. That's something the dogs key into right away and from there the connection is made and a relationship built. But children bring parents, relatives, carers and sometimes agencies ... someone responsible for the child. We are there to support any of these individuals and families (however constructed) who allow the dogs into their lives and so it is inevitable, that on the common ground of vulnerability, there might be a meeting of minds – and sometimes hidden heartache – where some time spent sharing the human-animal bond can help.

When Gracie Whitwam was admitted to the children's oncology ward the nursing staff thought of me. Gracie had acute myeloid leukaemia, the same as Ollie, so the thought was that if I spoke to her parents, I would be able to share my experience and perhaps ease their fears. I understood the request although it brought painful memories of my son's AML to the fore again. But then, I thought, would it have helped me if I had spoken to a parent who had been through the same experience? Yes, because empathy and understanding of a situation makes sense of everything. I told Gracie's parents that this, what was happening to them right then, was their 'new normal'. For as long as their child had leukaemia, they and Gracie's brother would feel like they were living with it too. That's just the way it is. All I could do was speak from experience; I knew what that 'new normal' was like with all its limitations. It was certainly the start of another long relationship with a family who, like all of us, would have done anything for their child not to be there, but I'm so glad that I was able to speak to them that day. And we were with Gracie the day she rang the End of Treatment Bell. What an amazing day that was for such a brave girl to celebrate such a massive milestone and a moment full of hope for a new start in life. I'm sure the dogs know the sound of that brass bell means laughter and plenty of hugs of 'thanks' for them.

As Gracie enjoyed many hours of laughter with Leo and friends, so too did 'Gorgeous' George O'Shaughnessy, who had a unique way of turning his relationship with leukaemia into a comedy sketch whenever possible. We had known George since he was two so we saw him grow up ... even in his first school uniform on the ward one time when he returned for an appointment. So often it was George who brightened our day as much as the dogs brought him smiles. George spent almost five years bouncing in and out of SCH and transferring to hospitals in Bristol and London for other treatment – which he never liked because then he would miss out on the therapy dog cards and stickers that he collected when he was with us. One thing George made sure that he never missed out on was the handing out of the Beads of Courage, which every child on the oncology ward are given – one for every procedure they have to go through. For long-term patients the length of threaded beads goes on and on for hundreds of metres. Maybe it's because I am an adult and a parent that I feel a certain sadness when I see a long string of the beads, but not children like George. To them the coloured beads are a badge of honour, a little victory over the monster cancer.

Of the thousands in his collection, George loved the paw-print beads – given for every visit from the dogs – best of all. Whenever we walked onto the oncology ward with Leo, or Karen went in with Archie, we would hear him call at the top of his voice: 'LOOK! It's the DOGS!!!' And when he was able, George would rush over and hug the dogs and tell everyone their names: 'This is Leo, he's my best friend'; other days it might be: 'This is Archie, he's my best friend!' The dogs didn't care and nor did the handlers; all we knew was that here was another little boy who loved the dogs and they loved him.

It was always extra fun if George was wearing one of his many dressing-up costumes and Leo was 'in disguise' too. They had great fun together! George was a big personality in a little guy and any down day could be brightened by his incredible spirit that I admired so much. He dealt with cancer by doing things that little children do: driving toy cars up and down the corridors, playing, painting, living life as normally and as fully as he could, despite being attached to drip lines and chemo paraphernalia.

When the RCN guidelines for 'Working with Dogs in Health Care Settings' was launched in May 2018, Gracie and George were featured in the media coverage. The *Mirror* captured some fabulous images of the children, accompanied by Leo and Archie, that said everything it's possible to say about what was being achieved with therapy dogs at SCH. It was right there – and we were once again happy to showcase what we were doing and what was possible. George, Gracie and the other patients who were pictured, were so happy to see themselves in the news and for me it was beyond all I could have hoped for. This was it. The launch of the guidelines was to take place at the RCN Congress in Belfast and I was flying out for the event.

It was the culmination of a lot of work with some incredible people for just over a year. When Amanda Cheesley had invited me to join the committee, I must admit that I had a massive bout of imposter syndrome at first, sitting with so many healthcare experts from so many different fields, but we soon realised that everyone had something to contribute to a protocol designed to make things safer and easier for all involved in AAI. I felt my role was to advocate for the dogs and handlers involved in it all. There were times when perhaps the clinical people around the discussion table might have wanted us to do more than we were able when working alongside an animal, so my part in some of the dialogue was me saying 'No!' Good job I had learned to say the word. Thanks to my Denver University studies I sat on the committee as the first person in Britain to earn the Certificate in Animal Assisted Therapy, Activities and Learning, and I felt I had a duty to be the advocate for doing things in the best possible way in healthcare.

When she invited me to attend the congress, Amanda also asked me to present the guidelines alongside her and Claire Pesterfield from the UK charity Medical Detection Dogs, who had her assistance dog Magic accompanying her. I took the first flight of the morning from Southampton and met Amanda and Claire at the conference centre in Belfast. It was very busy, lots of delegates walking around between the many rooms being used for the wide selection of lectures. Eventually, we found our way to where we needed to be and saw our lecture listed on the extensive programme.

We presented to a full lecture room, with people standing outside, craning their necks to see the huge screen; everyone wanted to hear the dog stories. We started with Claire talking about the importance of access rights for assistance dogs and – OMG, what an amazing dog – right in the middle of her talk, her dog Magic decided Claire needed more insulin, so interrupted her! I marvel at how clever he is and think of my dogs at home and realise they are just pet dogs with an exceptional role, nothing anywhere near as brilliant as Magic. Some may say that's not fair on my team – they are brilliant in a different way and lifesaving in some ways – but they are just not trained to be a diabetes medical alert assistance dog.

When it came to my turn, weirdly I wasn't really nervous even though I was speaking to a room full of people I'd never met before. I think the 'nerves' went out of me after Denver and because I was talking about my passion ... my dogs. That always makes public speaking so much easier. And this crowd of mainly health professionals looked a friendly lot. If I'm honest, a part of me was jealous of Claire having her dog beside her. I would have liked Leo to be there as he really is a great support to me when doing this kind of thing – radiating his calm. But as soon as I started talking and showing pictures of the children that have benefited from the presence of my therapy dogs, I felt myself filling with emotion and pride. I couldn't help it, it was just there. To be accepted into their young lives and give something through the support of a therapy dog at such a terrible and confusing time in their lives is, undeniably, a privilege.

Presentation finished, I saw a hand raised in the audience at the start of the Q&A. I didn't recognise the woman but what she said stunned me: 'I work at Southampton Children's Hospital and I just want to say I have seen the effects of Lyndsey and her team first hand. We as nursing staff have the benefit of what she has brought to the hospital and if anyone doubts what is being said, please don't. We see the responses whenever they are on the wards.' I could have burst! I was expecting a hand to go up and ask me something but not to be praised. I was genuinely taken aback and massively proud of the team all at the same time.

There were other questions to all of us and we answered them. However, I went away with that first comment ringing in my ears. I wanted to call Karen and Hannah right away to tell them what had been said, but as soon as Amanda closed our session, I was approached by senior nursing staff from four other hospitals who wanted me to consider helping them set up their therapy dog provision, which of course would be fabulous. I didn't want to burst their bubbles but I had to say that number-one priority must always be the right dogs in the hands of committed handlers with enough time to provide a service. I suspect we have made what we are doing at Southampton look easy because it's working so well. I appreciate every day that the type of commitment and availability we have between the handlers is not ordinarily achieved.

I chatted to some of the other delegates and then attended another presentation by Amanda on young adults' journeys through palliative care. That hit a nerve as the dogs have supported several young people through to end-of-life care: Jo and Alice being the first. I learned more from Amanda's presentation of the general lack of support and facilities for some families. I thought how sad that was because with the therapy dogs there is a warm and willing vehicle for supporting both patient and family, but of course that isn't the only thing these families need. The presentation was nothing to do with therapy dogs but every second I listened my inner voice said: 'That needs to be better ...' And even though I sometimes find it tough, I'm glad we are doing our little bit to support families like these when we continue to support patients who have chosen to have palliative care at home.

As I said my goodbyes, I realised I didn't feel great. I was exhausted, and when I arrived at Belfast airport I couldn't see properly. Shortly after that, I collapsed. When I came to, I was in the medical room, with everyone thinking I was a senior nurse as I was wearing a presenter badge from the RCN! I wasn't making much sense and they were concerned about whether I should fly. Truth is, I was simply exhausted, my adrenaline had drained away, I had a belting headache and I just needed to get home.

Much to my embarrassment I experienced more dizziness and collapsed again on the plane and they took me off and put me into an ambulance. When I came to, I persuaded them that I was perfectly compos mentis, despite the fact that at first I couldn't tell them the name of the prime minister or what year it was! I think they probably got a bit fed up with me saying that I was alright and wanted to go home, and as I had delayed the plane long enough, they decided to put me on it!

I don't think I could ever have been more relieved to get home to my family, our bed and, of course, the dogs. They were so pleased to see me and I told them I would tell them everything about the congress and launch and the person who said how wonderful they were ... tomorrow. It turned out that I had had a nasty migraine, the difficulty seeing and dizziness apparently common symptoms. I had experienced this only once before, many years earlier, but didn't know what it was, which was very scary. The ambulance team must have known when I came round, otherwise they would not have let me fly home. I am so pleased that they did. Perhaps they recognised I just needed sleep!

I was exhausted. Once more I had pushed the boundaries and this time, I pushed them a bit too far. I took it as a warning that without self-care, I would be no use to anyone or my beautiful dogs.

27

Passport to Animal Assisted Intervention

I CANNOT EXPLAIN THE JOY, EXHILARATION and relief I felt when our AAI received so much recognition after being on the television with Amanda Cheesley from the Royal College of Nursing. Suddenly, I realised we had come a very long way in just six years. Leo had been beside me the whole time and when I look at him, I see that it has been his own journey too.

Leo loving to be the centre of attention has been a real bonus from the day he joined me on this venture. When I say this, I'm including the range of TV interviews that we were invited to do at the time of the launch of the RCN guidelines. He was in great demand, not just for filming at hospital bedsides but also in television studios, where he always behaved perfectly and made me so proud. The thing is, because Leo is so good, I've always had to be careful not to over-work him. That's why, when a request for a late afternoon interview came in from our local station, ITV Meridian, I took Quinn along instead. Leo had been at work earlier in the day and Quinn was a youthful 17 months old, one of the team and qualified, so what could possibly go wrong? Apparently everything when I don't have enough sausages in my pocket to bribe him to stay on the seat next to me! Quinn decided that he would rather be away from the cameras and back in the green room with the nice folk who fed him biscuits ... thank you very much! It didn't matter, it made for a really funny set of out-takes and Leo had a rest from his celebrity duties. It just brought home to me that, in all of this, the dog's happiness has to be my priority and everyone around us must appreciate that's the way it has to be.

Entering the world of Animal Assisted Intervention was like suddenly being given an entry pass to a new planet where people want to meet and spend time with the dogs. Where there is a feeling that the canine magic is an aid to recovery or a last memory to ease an ending. I do feel the weight of responsibility in the task, but at the same time, I love it and I trust in the dogs, knowing that they just take it all in their stride. No more is asked of them than just being themselves.

And of course, where there is a dog, there can be laughter and they always make sure that smiles, for one reason or another, are on the cards. No matter how serious the mood or dire the diagnosis, they have the ability to transport patients out of their pain, anxiety, hospital boredom and reality.

And if all else fails ... there is always peanut butter!

Animal Assisted Therapy (AAT) is goal directed and outcome measured – something that we had to click into when we started to receive referrals from the clinical teams looking for a solution to a 'problem' – in our terms, an intervention with a therapy dog that provides a better way forward for the patient.

When I received this request from the play specialist on the paediatric medical unit (PMU) I had to smile ...

> Hi, we have a four-year-old boy. Non-verbal, he also has Down's syndrome. We have tried everything to get nasal prongs and Airvo on but no luck. I've been having a chat with Mum to get an idea of what he likes ... Not sure if you can help with Leo?

Little Sheylan had been through open-heart surgery and desperately needed to get used to wearing oxygen nasal prongs – a set of soft, flexible tubes that sit inside the nostrils – so he could receive the oxygen he so desperately needed to be able to go home. Unable to talk or understand what was being asked of him, I wondered if the way to reach our patient was to get Leo to look like he was wearing the prongs, for Sheylan to copy? His mum and I both had a set across our faces too. It was a game ... and the type that Leo plays best. Maybe he saw it as another kind of dress-up!

Sitting in front of a child where the only language we have is play and 'look at the dog', Leo was quite happy to be fussed by Sheylan and then let me drape the soft plastic prongs so they hung around the front of each nostril. We practised and it looked so much fun that Sheylan wanted to join in! I don't speak Romanian but there was plenty of communication with the boy's mum through Leo. And later, when she sent me a Facebook message and a photo of Sheylan wearing the prongs, I knew Leo had worked his magic again. Job done, and the patient could then be discharged.

It's when we do visits like that, I'm reminded of what we are really doing here. In his *Handbook of Animal Assisted Therapy*, Dr Aubrey Fine describes dogs as a 'social lubricant' because they connect with us without words. Communication does not need to involve the spoken word – sometimes it can't and sometimes confusion or fear blocks the ability to find the right words. That's when you need a therapy dog to just come in with an air of calm and silent understanding ...

Just like on one of the many days where we found ourselves heading for the paediatric orthopaedic ward to make a few visits, I heard a doctor say to the nurse that he would 'leave her to chat with Mum for a bit and come back in a while'. That was all I heard, but I wondered if there was something Leo could do to help. As it happened, we were visiting a patient in the next bed, so as the doctor left, pulling back the 'soundproof' hospital curtain, I saw a very upset and sad girl of about 9 years old, who had clearly worked herself up into a bit of a state about something.

She was giving her mum, the nurse and the doctor a difficult time because she didn't want her cannula put in, ready for her op. I had seen Leo comfort children like this many times, so I offered our help to the nurse, who checked with Mum that a dog visit was welcome and stepped in to assist. The nurse introduced us: 'This is Leo, he's the most popular member of our orthopaedic team when patients like you are nervous,' she said. With that, Leo sniffed the terrified girl's hands – they were shaking, she couldn't hold still. We chatted about her animals at home, her school, sibling, all the usual stuff, and in no time at all she had hopped off the bed and was sitting on the floor with her new flumpy friend, Leo. I could see that he was not for moving and quite happy to help.

The girl was due to have a small operation but she had already missed her scheduled slot on the list and I could see that the doctor was at the nurses' station, no doubt talking about potentially postponing the procedure. The nurse wondered if the doctor would be amenable to AAI support because then we could really help. It turned out he wasn't particularly keen on dogs, but as he could see the child was already distracted by Leo's snoozy ways – Leo was lying with his head in her lap – it was worth one last try.

I explained that Leo would lie close to her and all she had to do was look at him and bury her free hand in his coat and let the nurse hold her left hand – that way she wouldn't be able to see the cannula, she would only have eyes for Leo – and she agreed to try. I reassured her that Leo had helped lots of younger children with this so she was in safe paws. As I spoke, the nurse checked that the 'magic numbing cream' on her left hand was working and the girl gave Leo a treat with her free hand, which she then plunged into Leo's chest fur. 'OK,' I told her, 'he doesn't get another biscuit until we've finished! Now, just do some circling motions with your fingers so he thinks you're massaging him.' As Leo got a caring chest massage from his new friend, the doctor inserted the cannula and, thank goodness, the child's op was able to proceed. By this time, our young patient was last on the list instead of second – but it didn't matter because it was able to go ahead.

There was Leo, bridging the communication gap, making things possible, working his magic again.

When Liz and her golden retriever, Milo, joined the team I knew that we would be even more capable of keeping up with all the requests for our visits. We became four handlers and six dogs: Leo, Jessie, Quinn, Archie, Hattie, Milo. I felt guilty leaving out the pair I had started with, but Monty and Totty's retirements were well earned – after all, they had both, in one way or another, been my personal therapy dogs for years!

Having a larger team to offer support to the clinical teams meant that we could take therapy dogs onto the John Atwell Day Ward at SCH, where Archie was the poster-boy, showing children how having their pre-op checks, including blood pressure, temperature and pulse taken and chest listened to with a stethoscope, is not at all scary. Karen and Archie started to regularly see children on the day ward with autism, anxiety and learning difficulties who had upcoming procedures to see how Archie could help them. They would meet a couple of times informally before the big day, as part of the pre-op work up, with the play specialists prior to meds and then, if the clinical team thought it would help, they sometimes escorted their patient to theatre. Archie is chilled and confident and described in the hospital as a 'large mobile teddy bear' who seeks out cuddles. He shares his dad's temperament, so it's lovely to see that we almost have two Leos on the team!

With Liz and Milo we were further able to specifically help children who suffer from extreme anxiety, the kind that creates 'blocks' which hamper their treatment process. Milo is a big fan of Daniel and vice versa. Now aged 12, Daniel's mast cell activation disorder means that if he gets stressed, his immune system goes into overdrive, exacerbating the problem. It's important for Daniel to keep super-calm and the best way of doing that is with a dog supporting him, and he particularly loves having Milo as close to him as possible. It's not usual for therapy dogs to be allowed on the patient's bed: paws are fine on a waterproof pad, but with Daniel we have permission for Milo to join him on the bed so they can lie full-length together, cuddling up on a special protective sheet. It's such a wonderful thing to see, Daniel talking to Milo and soaking up the comfort as his anxiety levels reduce just before he is taken to theatre. Every time they meet it's like two best mates meeting up after a long time. He loves all of the dogs and of course we make sure that if Milo is off, one of the others supports him in the same way so we can still make what Daniel's mum calls magic ... and so do I.

After the launch of the RCN guidance and the media opportunities that it sparked, things started to hot up, in a good way, for the team. I started on this venture with Monty in 2013 and it wasn't long before we were invited onto the paediatric intensive care and oncology wards at SCH, but in the past few years our type of canine interaction with patients was no longer seen as 'unusual' but more as a beneficial aid. The therapy dog service was accepted and respected in a wider context as having huge potential.

Teenagers with physical and psychological illness, especially, responded so well to the presence of a therapy dog and the figures were starting to shout out loud too: we calculated that the therapy dog team had visited 2,500 patients in twelve months. That achievement did not go unnoticed and thank goodness we had a team in place to take up the additional requests that poured in.

That summer of 2018, I had never felt more grateful for my team, because life was just about to hurl some lemons.

On 20 July 2018, I discovered a lump in Totty's stomach. I asked Mike to double-check and he agreed with me, there was something there. I messaged Alex, our lovely vet, and she arranged for Totty to have a scan the following morning. We had travelled this same path twelve months earlier and that time we were lucky – the growth was operable and within a very short recovery time Totty was up and running with the youngsters, eager not to miss out on anything and acting as if nothing had ever happened. Even though this time she was eating and still very active, I was more worried.

Mike and I went to Alex's practice together. My gut instinct was that I didn't want to make the trip alone. As we watched Alex put the scanner on Totty's stomach, I held my breath in the hope that whatever was inside her could be removed, but Alex's face betrayed the truth: this second tumour was inoperable and it had affected her liver. Totty was given an injection of long-acting painkiller in case she was masking pain thanks to her stoical nature and we were ready to take her home and await Alex's call later to talk things through a bit more. Always our friend as well as our vet, she knew well enough that we, as a family, needed time to tell Harry and Ollie and for all of us to digest this news. I was so glad that we had the weekend ahead. Harry had always been very close to Totty, so I knew this would hit him hard. At least they had some time together to make a few more precious memories.

Totty was 11 years old, four years younger than Monty – this wasn't supposed to happen to her yet. Strange, but when we got home, I noticed the other dogs were treating her differently … What did they know? I felt sure they had been acting normally around her until we had gone to the vets, but now they were sniffing and moving around her, as if giving her space but curious to know why she had been out of the house. How did they know? Maybe her 'smell' changed to them and I was only just noticing. Could they detect the difference in her, as the Medical Detection Dogs who are trained to sniff out various cancers and conditions such as diabetes and serious illnesses such as malaria and Covid-19. It was as if, to them, she was no longer the original Totty … as they knew her.

That same afternoon my brother called to ask if I had heard from Mum about Dad. I told Kieran that I hadn't: 'Well, Dad went for a scan earlier and it appears that he doesn't need a knee replacement, he has a massive tumour in his buttock and it's likely a sarcoma.' How does that happen to two members of my family in one day? Totty and Dad both had sarcomas.

It was so hard to take in. Maybe I didn't really want to take it in because accepting it would make it real. My dad had been limping for a while and I had been nagging at him to get his joints checked. He had suddenly been taken ill the day before with chest pains but the X-rays showed little, so they decided to do a scan and include other areas. I knew nothing of all of this that was going on in Bournemouth, and Mum and Dad knew nothing about what was happening to Totty. My dad had gone to the radiology department from the ward on a trolley and apparently said he would struggle to lift his leg up to get onto the scanner. The very kind radiographer called one of the doctors, who requested additional scans to include the appropriate parts. Just as well she did – there on the scan was a huge tumour. I was devastated to the point of numbness.

Totty crossed the rainbow bridge a week later, by which time she had stopped eating and had a small amount of blood in her stools. She was put to sleep at home, and before Alex arrived, I baked a batch of heart-shaped cakes, iced and topped with ham and sardines (toppings chosen to ensure I wouldn't be tempted to eat them!) and then spent some special time with Totty on her own in the garden. She had her last meal when Alex arrived and despite not having eaten for a day, she gulped down the cakes with the others looking on through the gate of their pen.

Totty died in her favourite place just opposite the kitchen window, leaning against the wall where she liked to look down the garden. The others watched from about ten feet away, probably wondering what on earth was going on. I'm sure they were really confused by it all, being kept separate in the main garden and the tempting treats they could smell but couldn't reach. And who knows, maybe they sensed an ending. I don't know.

When Totty had passed, I opened the gate and her daughter Jessie rushed in, sniffed the plate on the floor and went straight out again! Through my tears I couldn't help but smile – I suspected that she just wanted to check for any leftover cakes. Monty came in, put his head down and gave Totty a nuzzle before coming to my side. Leo just came straight to me, looking a little confused, not really knowing what to do. Jessie returned to be with us once she had picked up a toy to bring us once her brain had switched from food to the severity of the situation. We took all of them into the main garden and played a little bit, but their energy was low, so I just let them take in what was happening, if that's what they wanted to do, while I waited for the pet undertaker to arrive.

Totty looked so beautiful, serene and peaceful now the pain had gone. I could see the puppy in her again, and the dog who loved to run with me and lie in her favourite place stretched out in the sun. I kissed her and Alex kissed her as we hugged. I really valued Alex's friendship, especially at that time, as Mike and the boys were not around that day. I was left thinking my thoughts about the lovely puppies Totty had given to us over the years and what a good mother she had been to all of them. And she had given us Jessie, who was a star in her own right. It was hard to take in that Totty had gone.

Once I was alone, I put the leads on the dogs and took them round the block for a quick walk ... Well, I say a 'quick' walk, it was really a short walk done at Monty's slow pace. At almost 15 years old, he was in no hurry to go anywhere but he did like to go out on a plod and let everyone know he was still around. The following day we carried on with our normal routine: out with Monty for his little stroll, then Leo, Jessie and Quinn for a longer off-lead country walk and then back for their breakfast. The routine kept us all in check and kept my big emotions under control. As I drank my cup of tea, I thought about Totty who had a life of never being left behind in the slow lane, unlike old Monty. She always kept up with the younger ones in the pack at all times and it made me wonder what dogs would prefer, if given the choice: to go before you have to endure the trappings of old age or stay the course until infirmity grinds you to a halt?

I didn't allow myself to have many more feelings about Totty as thoughts of my dad took over. He looked terrible and my brother and sister-in-law, who are both doctors, together with Mike, were not sounding particularly hopeful. Sarcomas like dad's do not have a good outcome. I managed my grief for Totty and kept going. I walked the dogs, did some hospital visits, worked on my business and then very quickly found myself organising a big family lunch to create some memories with my brother's family and ours. Mum and Dad, with their son and daughter's families all together, a chance for lots of photographs to be taken while Dad could still stand. The following week he couldn't, so our big family lunch had happened in the nick of time.

The first two weeks, Dad appeared shell-shocked by the diagnosis but at least he was able to get out and about, then it all became very different as he soon became immobile due to the rapid growth of the tumour and his overall strength drained. Just four weeks later the disease took him, Dad left us ... it was true, he had a really aggressive, inoperable sarcoma. I felt lost and reached out to my hobby to carry me through. I found I wanted to visit the patients, I needed to carry on with the AAI and my dogs to take me to my happy place through all the trauma. Mike had work to do, of course, and for much of the time I found myself alone with my thoughts and the dogs. Our sons were grieving for their grandfather too and there were times where we all needed to be together and other times when we just needed to do our own thing. It was a tough time for everyone.

Fellow handlers Karen, Liz and Hannah as well as Joyce, who oversees our team as youth and play services manager, knew what was going on, but not the staff nor the patients, which meant I was able to keep up my visiting without being asked about what was happening in my life. The day before and the day after my dad's funeral, Leo and I went into intensive care to see a child ... No one knew why it made such a difference to me. I needed to be there with Leo, doing what we do. I had to keep going.

There was another reason I had to keep my distress buried deep – the contents of a letter that arrived the day after we lost Totty. With everything going on I'd pushed the post to one side but this was one I should have opened right away. It was informing me that a routine mammogram had found something and I needed to go for a biopsy. I cursed and wondered what on earth was going to be thrown in our direction next ... and then I called Mike.

While taking the biopsy, they decided that they could go ahead and remove the little lump that was there, which they did under ultrasound guidance with local anaesthetic … and then I drove myself home. If only I could have taken Leo in with me, I feel sure I would have been so much calmer. Thankfully, seventy-two hours later my results were in and I had confirmation that it was benign. I could forget all about it – phew!

A few weeks later, when the pet undertaker called to say that Totty's ashes were ready for collection, I drove over to Fair Oak to bring her home. That was my time to break. To let the emotion loose and start to grieve, because everything with Dad and Totty was scrunched inside me like a ball clogged in my chest. I had to let some of it out. I sat on the floor hugging Jessie – her firstborn – and cried into her coat. I cried, while everything about this one normally described as our busy-bodied 'floofy' girl was so very calm. She put her head in my lap and we sat together remembering her mum. I looked at Monty lying in the middle of the lounge floor and said to him: 'I thought that you would be first to say goodbye, old fella … I'm glad you're still here for us.'

I didn't report Totty's death on social media. I am not one for long lists of condolences or sympathy and most important to me is that I want our Animal Assisted Intervention *Leo & Friends Therapy Dogs* and the new *SCH Therapy Dogs* pages to be happy, upbeat places for parents and clinical teams to share their stories and drop into and out of as they like. On my own personal Facebook page, I posted that my dad had gone to walk Totty … and my friends knew what I meant by that.

There is a design fault in dogs. I think we should get them when the time is right for us and they should live until we go. Then we would grow old together. In every other respect, they are perfect.

28
Watching over me

I GUESS IT WAS JUST HOW THE YEAR was panning out, but when we were asked to visit a leukaemia patient, Ben Walker, once again I wondered if my experiences would help his family. Each request to see an AML patient reminded me of the worst times from a decade earlier. A time when we wondered initially 'Why us?' but soon came to think 'Why not us?' Cancer doesn't discriminate ... it happens to such a mix of families, sadly. He was 10 years old and I thought immediately of Ollie, which was ironic because Ben soon said he wanted to meet someone who had survived this horrid journey. I spoke to my son knowing that it was a big ask and again assured him that he was not part of my payback promise – that was mine alone. Ollie happily agreed to pop in one evening as guests of his parents and talk to Ben. So, there we were with our patient, me, Ollie and, this time, Jessie getting all the fuss.

I know Ollie knew what it was like from Ben's perspective. He didn't have to agree, but he did and I was so proud of him and Jessie, just sitting there being herself, all wide-eyed and with tail wagging.

We attended Ben's funeral the following year and it was heart-breaking. Leo had seen Ben several times so he accompanied me and Ollie took Jessie. The dogs had been invited and were there to comfort the family, who looked as happy to see them there as they had always been delighted to see them at Ben's bedside. On that day I felt grateful, I felt so fortunate; this could have been my situation.

Bereavement. I am no expert, but having lost my dad and other close relatives, I know something about losing older people. Thankfully, I have no personal knowledge of losing a child to ill health or accident. What I do know is that I think this phrase that is attributed to HM The Queen Mother, who mourned the loss of her husband HRH King George VI, fits well for everyone: 'Grief doesn't get better, you just get better at it.' I have mentioned this to some of the parents along the way in the hope that it will help them as it helped me. It also resonates for the parents hiding their feelings while supporting their children through life-affecting health issues. I believe that you are also entitled to grieve for the carefree life you had before a major illness. I know there were times when Ollie was ill, and even well after he had been treated, that I yearned not to have a nagging worry in my head. I describe it as like a blue sky with one cloud in it ... as long as the cloud stays away, everything will be OK. But I know that I am so fortunate only to have experienced the level I have.

It's not always easy to recognise when you need to bring professional help into your life but I was glad that I took the opportunity to speak to a clinical psychologist working with children on the oncology ward at Southampton when Ollie was a patient. At that time, I was not especially good at opening up to her when she popped her head around the door and I must have seemed pretty resistant to talking to her. Later, once Ollie had been discharged, we arranged a family meeting for all of us, thinking it would be good for the boys. We hadn't anticipated it would be us adults who got the most out of it, finally realising that our coping strategies had gone and we needed some time to make sense of what had happened to us.

When I returned to SCH, now as a volunteer, I saw the same clinical psychologist on the ward and over time I recognised some parents were in the same place that I'd been – coping but not really coping. So, I shared my own experience with many of them, both in relationship to me as a mother and our family in general, including the role of Harry the sibling. On many occasions I have been able to persuade parents that there is a benefit to having a chat with the professional on hand or to encourage their child's sibling to do so. It's good to know that there is help out there and how good it can be to invite an expert into your armoury.

Occasionally I still find myself needing some support. I was in tears when I spoke to the expert because I felt so wretched for a cared-for child who was in hospital at the same time as Ollie. I had watched him coveting his time playing with Ollie and chats with the staff or other parents so much, because he had no family with him. His support workers would be there sometimes and occasionally a friend would come in, but he had nowhere near the support every other child had on the oncology ward. Life did not just give that boy lemons, it gave him a lemon grove, and I will admit it made me angry for a while. A few years later his new carer family contacted me via social media and asked if I could help them put together some memories for the boy, including his oncology journey. He was no longer in touch with anyone else who had been caring for him at the time he was on the ward. I spent a few hours collating those precious hospital memories for him and it was great to be able to share them with the boy and Ollie when they met again after so long. Memories are so important and so very special. Now I often talk about us creating memories using AAI, he was one of the patients who inspired me to make sure every patient we meet creates memories on their hospital journey. Those memories will be a mix of good, bad, sad and hilarious and, with a therapy dog, there will likely be lots of smiles from captured priceless moments.

I was happy to see the end of 2018 from a family perspective because it will forever, in my memory, be associated with the great losses of my dad and Totty. We have so many photographs of them both to ensure that they will live on with us ... forever.

On the flip side, the year saw our therapy dogs become even more accepted and requested for duty within SCH. I was living something I had dared to dream and I had my friends and golden dream-makers at my side. Totty is still looking down the garden from her favourite spot, maybe looking to see if one of those sardine-topped cakes is there to be sniffed out. Whenever I see a rainbow, I imagine she is there watching over us.

Part Four:

Going for Golden

29

Love and loss

I REMEMBER THAT NAGGING VOICE that I heard so clearly at the start of this journey of mine: 'What have you got to be down about? You have a loving husband, two gorgeous boys and a lovely home ... pull yourself together, woman!' In those days I was good at presenting a happy front to the world while inside my head there was sometimes a lonely void hollowed out by dark thoughts and bouts of self-doubt and depression. That was until a wonderful, life-changing thing happened to get me off my self-destructive mental merry-go-round – I invited a dog into my life.

Fate, in its weird and wonderful way, I think, took over from there. It took me by the hand and dragged me into Southampton Children's Hospital with Ollie as a patient with a 65 per cent chance of making it. I lived the life of the hospital parent and discovered what I had imagined to be true, was true. Life in hospital is not an easy one – but a dog is a wonderful distraction, a therapy and a familiar reminder of home and normality. It's something good to hold onto – physically and emotionally. Nowadays, Leo and the team prove, every single day they are on duty, that there can be a magical connection between a dog and a child.

When I made a deal with myself that night in the hospital in 2008, I had no idea where it would take me. I had no idea how I was going to give back at that point; I just knew I had to. Whatever fearful presence was with me in that midnight moment on the stairs, it held me in its grip – and, I admit, it still does. Once cancer has crashed into your life, it never really leaves, and the drive to give back when your child has escaped its clutches is huge. Fear drove me at first, as if Satan himself was on my back, urging me through every painful mile of those fundraising marathons.

And then fate helped me find the pathway ahead and the partners who were to join me on this mission – my dogs. I could not have chosen better allies to accompany me – not because they can't answer back but because they have the three basic ingredients for its success: empathy, trust and innate kindness.

'Without the insecurities I wouldn't be where I am now.' I heard pop star Robbie Williams say that in the Happy Place Podcast where he was talking to presenter Fearne Cotton (December 2020). I echoed the words out loud: 'But isn't that me too?' My mission to take Animal Assisted Intervention to SCH was only made possible by my dogs. Without Leo's special canine traits that some would call insecurities – his neediness, demand for cuddles and constant reassurance – he would not have been the dog to partner me in taking this so far and to so many people, to so many sick children. He is, as I've said, my partner in care. From a puppy Leo 'spoke' to me in a way that told me he was different.

He wasn't Monty, the big, solid, teddy, protector-type, ready to catch me when I fell emotionally – which I did many times in the dark times – and he saved me. Instead, Leo saw something in me that 'fitted' with something in him. We both needed someone to lean on, I needed someone to consistently have my back, to make up that missing measure of confidence I needed to step into a room full of people, to be present with parents reeling from their child having a devastating accident or difficult prognosis. And I think I felt in him his need for protection, love, reassurance. I always say that Leo is a 'leaner', but in reality, we lean on each other, physically and emotionally.

We are each other's glue.

He attempts to be with me all the time, and when he decides that I must touch him, he will ensure that I do – if I'm typing, he pops up under my arm so his head is between my hands! He has to share me when the other dogs are around but on hospital visits, he has me all to himself – we are a double act. We complement each other. From the first day I took him into children's intensive care I saw him tune in to the patients with a kind of canine sixth sense. His expression says: 'How can I help you?' His easy body language says: 'I'm here for you.' And if that isn't the essence of the human-animal bond at work, I don't know what is. We are a partnership and it's Leo who has walked the therapy path most closely with me. I owe him so much – for being, simply, him.

The trouble with having such a close bond with a dog is

that when they leave you it is utterly devastating. We lost Monty on 11 March 2019. He had been physically doddery for a while but always his lovely, happy self. As long as he could see me, he was absolutely fine. If he couldn't see me, he let out a single bark to 'ask' where I was. The beginning of the end was a rare evening when Mike and I were sitting together watching something on the television, all the dogs relaxed around us. When the time came to get them on their feet and head for bed, Monty just couldn't get up. He looked so helpless. I stayed with him overnight in the lounge and he slept OK, but I think, in my heart, I knew this was the time.

The following morning, he still couldn't stand and his eyes seemed less able to follow me. I called our vet Alex to tell her how Monty was and we both knew how this would end, so we arranged for her to come to us later. My friend Carole came round to see him. She adored the old boy, and he loved her too, but this time his expression was vacant. By the time Alex arrived, poor Monty could barely recognise her. Usually, he was full of bounce as he greeted her, but not this time. I made him the same sardine-topped cakes that I had made Totty before she crossed the rainbow bridge and he dutifully ate them but he had so little energy; he was so very, very tired. It was as if he had seen Mike home and the two of us finally relaxing together, just the two of us, and he knew his job was done.

It was a time when I needed to draw breath in my hectic life and I think Monty knew that, and knew that if he went that particular day, I would not be alone as Mike was with me. Monty was the most amazing dog. He was the first of my golden partners and such a good reason for having five. To help me cope with the heartache I wrote a eulogy:

Monty ...

My friend, kindness mentor, psychologist and exercise partner has retired from my life.

Monty has known me
Happy and sad
Calm and angry
Healthy and sick
Fat and thin
Optimistic and pessimistic
Judgemental and non-judgemental
Frantically busy and relaxed

At work, home and on holiday, his love has never wavered.

This furry companion was eternally loyal, knew me better than I knew myself, loved me like I was his world, he knew me and stood by me longer than some of my human friends did.

Took it to heart when I left him for a few days and pined but never bore a grudge and was elated when I returned.

When Mike and I celebrated our silver wedding anniversary I had, on paper, spent 25 years with him but, thanks to Mike's career, the reality was I'd spent much more time with Monty, who was 14 at the time.

I owe this boy my life, my outlook on life and all that is canine in my life ... If he had not been the dog he was there would only ever have been one and my world would have been poorer for it.

Losing loved ones is part of life – we all know that – and sadly an inevitable part of our role at Southampton Children's Hospital. It is maybe a part of what we do that doesn't come immediately to mind because when you imagine working with the beautiful, crazy mix of children and dogs, whatever the environment, it has all the promise of being so much fun! It is fun ... and at the same time it can on occasion be so incredibly, horribly, heartbreakingly sad.

The loss of a child is a loss that a family carries with them forever. A Christmas marred forever, a birthday celebrated without the birthday boy or girl. It is a lingering shadow and why many funerals are styled as a celebration, which means that we are often invited to attend, because the dogs have become a fun and comforting part of the child's end-of-life care and final memories for their loved ones.

When we lost 'Gorgeous' George that summer in 2019, it was a sadness that came at the end of almost five years of Leo and the rest of the therapy dog team being in the life of this incredibly brave soul. George was only two years old when he first met Leo on the children's oncology ward and from then on leukaemia had kept him on an invisible rubber band, constantly pulling him between home and hospital, where Leo, Archie, or whoever was George's assigned 'best mate', was always popping in for a visit. Amy, George's mum, said to me one day: 'The dogs bring a sense of normality to a very abnormal and scary situation and so much joy.' And for George's sister, Bella, Leo was a playmate when she visited, and so many family photographs have Leo or Archie or both of them central to the action.

It was the same at the celebration of George's life. Bella came over to sit between Leo and Archie, cuddling them as she watched the video of her big brother and the therapy dogs enjoying fun times together to the end. Karen and I looked at each other and then we ourselves needed to seek comfort by stroking our dogs as we looked at Bella sitting between them. There were so many children there and the dogs became a focus of attention for them, and a few of the adults too – that's the thing with dogs, they don't need you to say the 'right' words or do the 'right' thing in awkward situations because they are just there for you in the moment. The children took stickers from us to remember the day and sat with Leo and Archie for emotional support.

It was, as always, a heart-breaking privilege to be invited to join a family at their darkest time and I'm sure the dogs feel it too. They are always calm and extremely giving at funerals. For many youngsters they will never have been to one before and lots have no idea what to say ... so, all the time, they talk about the dog. I know Leo is at his calmest at funerals as if he knows automatically exactly what is expected of him. I look at him and think how Harry and Ollie have so many nicknames for Leo, far more than any of our other dogs. I think their description of him being as 'soft as creamy French cheese' is pretty apt because he is a gooey, sensitive soul and that's why I have to be sure to protect him in situations where he can become the focus of so much emotional attention.

It's not unusual for a family to request we sit close at a funeral, very often in the row directly behind them, which I always hope doesn't upset people who have known the family way longer than we have. Leo, for instance, always settles quickly and I think senses what will happen next. It doesn't take long before a hand from one of the parents or siblings reaches back to stroke the dog for comfort. I try so hard to lock away my own emotion for the time we are needed because if I let that moment get to me, I'll be lost. Tears gather when I see a parent's hand caressing the dog's fur where their child's hand had once done the same.

Another good friend of the dogs who had starred in our ward Christmas video became an angel in early 2019. The therapy dogs had been such a fun part of Keira's life for three years in and out of SCH. Leo has a habit of reaching in and finding what it is that his patients need from him – and in Keira, he found a girl sometimes deep in thought but also so ready to come out of her shell, eventually taking part in the Christmas video and other photocalls with the dogs and making memories along the way. She had become very close to Leo and Archie on our visits to the oncology ward, so we visited her together as she was cared for at home during her palliative phase.

You can't simply walk away from a family that has welcomed Leo and his friends into their lives. Visiting the children in hospital is one thing, but to continue to visit and be part of their palliative care at home is a no-brainer if that is what they want. Whenever we are requested to visit, I know that we're not really just 'visiting'; we are guests of people hurting. Many are just about coping with the hell that has descended on them and the challenge of fitting the stresses of normal life and work around the care of their child. At the front door of one of these homes there is nothing to betray the pain inside. Neat flower borders, bright, tidy hall and walls covered in family photographs dating from happier times, comfy living room with books and flowers; normal life that has been invaded by a hospital bed and medical paraphernalia. The mixing of the lives, the past and the present, the before and after. I see all of that when I'm invited into a home; I can dip into my own fears but Leo does not. He cuts through all of that to see only the poorly child to comfort and the sadness to put on hold for everyone present if only for the time that he is there.

Palliative care can be a heartbreakingly tough for someone in the advanced stages of their illness and their wider family. How difficult it must be to live with such a big shadow lurking, even when you hope with every fibre of your being that a medical solution may be found. I always think of that when I visit, as I did when I took Leo to see 11-year-old Brooke Leavey at home, which is just a stone's throw from my own. In that short distance a different family life was being lived and all I knew from social media and the local news reports was of fundraising efforts to help send Brooke to the States for treatment as she had been living with DIPG (diffuse intrinsic pontine glioma), a cruelly aggressive type of childhood cancerous tumour that forms in the brain stem affecting most basic functions in the body, from breathing to talking, walking and hearing. Leo and I had seen Brooke on the wards not long after she was diagnosed and saw her again for the first time in a while, quite by chance, on a day Leo was doing his rounds dressed in his doggy Harry Potter outfit (plus spectacles). She was so happy when we were asked to go into her room. Happier still when I helped Leo to rest his paw on her bed. Brooke reached out and touched his fur and in that second, phone cameras flashed around as the family called to Leo to look their way so they could capture those precious smiles.

I walked away thinking how glad I was that people could just ask us to pop in like that. That we could be there in the moment for Brooke and her family. They needed that visit and I was pleased to be following up with her at home, with the blessing of the oncology outreach nursing team who were looking after her palliative care. Leo, in his famous lion wig, brought smiles to all the faces in the room. He was there for everyone, not Brooke alone, in the saddest of times. Brooke Maria Leavey, always a bright star who loved to sing, dance and entertain and who loved the showman in Leo, lost her fight for life on 14 March 2020. She will be remembered as forever beautiful and forever 11 years old.

Lots of people ask me how I feel about the journey I take with the therapy dogs and the children. I don't think I can be there for the children and their families during the fun smiles on the wards without also supporting them if they want us through the tough stuff. Of course, I would prefer all the children made a recovery and everyone lived happily ever after, but life isn't like that sadly. It is a two-sided coin: on the one side we have the great joy of sharing some memories that are quirky, funny and inspirational, while on the other there are memories that make your heart ache for the children and families involved. It is no different for the professional staff at the hospital. Thankfully as a team we always have someone to talk to. Karen, Hannah, Liz and I know when one of us has been supporting a family having a tough time and we are there for each other to talk to and to decompress.

As an aside, this was one of the things added to both the Royal College of Nursing addendum to high-risk areas in 2019 and the Intensive Care Society guidelines I helped write more recently – that AAI handlers encounter some situations that they may need to talk about afterwards to decompress and they should be offered the same occupational health support as the salaried staff are in hospitals. We can access it at Southampton and Donna always contacts me to ask me if I'm OK if she knows I have experienced a challenging case in intensive care. If I have, my first thought is to hug the dogs a bit tighter and thank them for being there. Leo never minds that, he is always ready for an extra hug. The next time we go in, we may just be faced with smiley meet-and-greet, the easy Animal Assisted Activity, but that's just the way we love it ... a mix of all aspects of AAI, from the easy 'hellos' to the more emotionally challenging relationships.

30
Being there

I REMEMBER 2019 AS A WHIRLWIND of speaking engagements and conferences. I kept telling myself that it would all calm down soon but I wasn't convincing myself at all. I was grateful for Sally, my loyal colleague, who would sort out things in my business while I was out doing AAI stuff. Thank goodness she was there at times as things just got so busy. I am sometimes reminded of the time I was asked how I felt about coordinating a region for the Pets As Therapy charity and just the thought of it was too much: 'I'm sorry,' I said, 'I don't even have the time to coordinate an outfit some days, never mind anything else!' And here I was again.

At the National Association of Play Specialists Conference in London, I was captivated by a talk delivered by a child psychiatrist at Great Ormond Street Hospital. He asked the audience if anyone had or has had a mental health issue. Only about half the audience indicated that they had; I was one of them. He implied that the rest of the audience were hiding something as everyone has mental health *and* physical health issues. It's all a balance and I knew that he was right. He next put up a slide which had a quote from the World Health Organization: '*Mental health is defined as a state of wellbeing in which every individual realises his or her own potential can cope with the normal stresses of life, can work productively and fruitfully and is able to contribute to his or her community.*' I empathised with that totally. Although functioning, I was still very aware that we are all a living balancing act.

Joyce, our youth and play services manager, and I had a talk to give that day, but this talk was one that really hit home. We are all likely to tell ourselves that we are OK, that we are coping and there's nothing wrong, when in reality it may not be true. I attended that talk just at the right time to remind me that I needed to remember the importance of self-care. To accept that I would be of no use to anyone if I took on too much and flaked out again.

Thankfully, there were engagements at which I could include the team, to take the pressure off. When we attended the annual PIER (Paediatrics Innovation Education and Research) conference in Southampton a few months later, where we had both a poster and verbal presentation accepted, I presented with Donna, the advanced purse practitioner from PICU – and then looked forward to relaxing with the team – but first a photograph with the dogs. Leo was already on the podium with me when we checked our PowerPoint talk was set to run OK, and when Milo and Archie joined us for the line-up, they were really excited to be the centre of attention. Standing in front of the one-metre-high illuminated letters, PIER, Milo gave a swift swish of his tail and ... the letter R went off the back of the podium! That was it ... we were at the PIE conference!

Dogs spark humour wherever they go and I believe that's where the balance is achieved. We try to move too fast and the dogs remind us that we need to slow it down. I trust their judgement – they are never wrong. I took it as a warning to take it easy and, if I was taking it easy, maybe it was a good time to invite another puppy into the Uglow pack.

Catherine called me from France to say that she had a special puppy for me – if I wanted a puppy that was! We talked about it and I decided that I should go and see the litter, which of course meant I was going to have one. Catherine knew that if I was going to continue taking therapy dogs into the hospital, I would soon need another puppy, especially now that Jessie was nine and Leo eight years old, with Quinn just two years old.

As ever, it was Joker, Leo's father, who greeted me like a long-lost friend when I arrived at Catherine's home and took me to see Millie and her pups. Like a proud elder statesman, Joker had to be in on it. It's easy to see where Leo's people-loving personality comes from.

The new puppy, Pollyanna, and her litter mates were in the garden. She was beautiful, of course, and looked very confident playing with her siblings. When I cuddled her, the little golden bundle felt perfect in my arms. Catherine had chosen her – but then she had chosen me too, and Leo. I'm never good at waiting, but it's part of taking on a puppy and, if I'm honest, part of the excitement too! I had to leave Pollyanna to return home and wait until she could be passported to come to the UK.

* * *

There was enough to do while I was waiting for our new arrival and I had a promise to keep. Bella, Gorgeous George's sister, was starting school in September and I wanted to take Leo to see her when she came out after her first day. Support for families like George O'Shaughnessy's does not always end at the hospital or on the day of the funeral. My thought was that we could be there to support her, as George would have done if he could have been there. Leo always made a fuss of her and I was sure that he would feel the need to give double-fuss when we met her. Bella was so happy to see Leo at the gate to give her a cuddle and she was soon telling her new teacher and friends who he was. She was sad and happy all at the same time and it took me back to what she said at George's celebration of life, where she spent the whole time with Leo and Archie: 'I love seeing the dogs because they are so beautiful and cuddly and make me feel happy.'

Therapy dogs filling gaps in children's lives is maybe where they reign supreme. Perhaps if Leo had been born out of a fur coat his career would have taken him into healthcare or social work because, like me, he has an eye for the underdog. I remember thinking this when we met Emily White, a teenager with spina bifida whose anxiety went off the scale whenever she had to attend hospital appointments and especially when she faced surgery. Emily's autism made her particularly sensitive to stressful situations but when she met Leo, everything changed. Leo must have keyed into this 14-year-old's vulnerability because he just moved in for a cuddle and he got one right back! Emily's mum told me: 'Leo and Quinn are so cuddly and now when Emily needs a procedure she can just stroke them while it's happening and she is so calm. Having the dogs there has changed everything for her and for me, as I can get a sneaky cuddle too.' When I hear words like this I know that we are truly there for a reason and in a role that only a dog can fill.

So very often the look on a child's face lets you know that a visit from the dogs is the highlight of their day. When Rosina was on the oncology ward the dogs were her favourite visitor. She was being treated at the same time as waiting for all the red tape to be sorted in order for her carer family to be finalised, and in the meantime, Leo and his team were happy to go some way to fill that big gap for a very poorly teenager.

Rosina had a brain injury caused by her cancer which sometimes made her forgetful and occasionally have angry outbursts, but seeing Leo in all his various costumes was her calming therapy; even when she was having her chemotherapy or in a period of enforced medical isolation, she was able to see us through the window. She was on the ward at a time when, Tate, another big fan of ours, was in isolation. Tate and Leo had perfected the 'high five for isolated patients' routine at the window, whereby the dog's paw 'touched' the patient's hand from the other side of the glass and the smiles would come despite not being able to feel the fur.

When it all became clear that Rosina's days were running short, all the dogs including Leo, Jessie, Quinn, Milo, Archie and Hattie took it in turns to see her every day to support this special patient at her most challenging time. Nearing the end of her life, it was her birthday, and having seen Leo and the others in the preceding days it was Quinn who came to visit, carrying a birthday card with a big 'R' in paw prints on the envelope. Seeing us arrive and knowing things were changing quickly now, Rosina's consultant granted Quinn special permission to lie next to her on her bed on a protective mat. She hugged him tight before asking me if she could give me a hug. I lifted Quinn back onto the floor and, with the blessing of her social worker who was with us, I leant in to receive the hug that Rosina so wanted to give. She held on and whispered 'thank you' in my ear. As the hug ended, I turned to look at Quinn who, even with his lead over my wrist, had managed to crane his neck up to the tray table and was ... busy licking her birthday cake! Horrified, I turned to Rosina and apologised ... she laughed out loud and told me it had come from Marks & Spencer in the hospital foyer, so I rushed downstairs to buy another with my naughty dog who was trying really hard to lick the thick cake icing out of the roof of his mouth!

The smiles when Rosina had her wish come true to hold my new pup Pollyanna made everyone around her cry, me included. I had already seen so much of this period in end-of-life care, this easing away to know that, if permitted, it was vital to grant an achievable final wish. Pollyanna was the last dog Rosina saw. It brought so much happiness and peace to a girl who simply loved the dogs. As time slipped away, I messaged Rosina's carers to offer support: 'If, and when, you think it's appropriate, tell her that Monty and Totty are waiting to be her therapy dogs up in Heaven.' And indeed, Rosina had that comfort before she '... simply didn't breathe again.'

At the funeral, Archie and Milo were there to support Rosina's family and friends, including her mother and siblings, just as the dogs had instinctively given Rosina solace and smiles in hospital.

I know the dogs felt her passing was close. As each of them left her for the last time over her final few days, it was as if they knew. Karen said that the day before Rosina's birthday, Archie wanted to go back into Rosina's room. As they turned to leave, he was pulling to go back in.

31
Counting my blessings …

LIKE THE CHANGING SEASONS THAT I SEE on my daily dog walks, I know that all events, good and bad, must pass and learning to live with each of the big changes can be close to impossible. As some of our friends become our angel friends, I can't help hugging my own sons a little closer every time I see them and being grateful for all I have. That's what drives me to see what else we can do to bring some fun and reassurance to the children in SCH. The arrival of Pollyanna in our home gave me a view to the future.

Harry and I went to collect her from France and, again, it was an emotional goodbye from Catherine and her family. Clearly, Pollyanna had carved a place in their hearts, just as Leo had, and once she was home and running in the garden it was plain to see that she was a chip off the old block. Jessie, Leo and Quinn welcomed her with a big sniff and that was that! But I think Quinn took a while to work out that he was no longer the baby of the family. As Jessie and Leo's son he was used to that role, but I think he decided that he'd be better placed in the ranking as

Pollyanna's big brother and so he happily stepped into those new shoes – although I wasn't entirely sure that our new girl needed a male lead. She was on first sight sassy, brainy, pretty, had a fabulous golden coat and very dark eyes that stared into you. Her features are finer than Jessie's – I'd say that she has a touch of the glamour girl about her. Not only that, but being the youngest she also always gets the toy she wants, the bed she wants, everything, because she is queen bee of the pack and so clever. Leo isn't bothered by any of it. My boy is more 'anything for a quiet life'.

I watch Pollyanna play and wonder what adventures she'll get up to when she reaches her time to come to work on the wards. She started well with that highly emotional visit to Rosina, and then not long after to Emily Jones, another girl receiving palliative care treatment but this time at her home. She too wanted to meet the new dog in our pack and it was a pleasure to grant her that wish.

Looking back, we've had some great times. I remember one of the early days visiting with Leo I was on the paediatric intensive care ward to see a patient and one of the consultants thanked me afterwards for being there. He said that the emotional lift our visits gave to the staff on his unit was incredible, only matched by the annual visit from the Southampton football team! That comment stayed with me and then when I was studying for my AAI qualification, I came across a quote in one of my textbooks: 'An indirect way to improve patient care is to improve the mood of the staff. The benefits that dogs bring into an environment are not limited to the people receiving care; they also extend to the people providing care.' (K. Butler, *Therapy Dogs Today*.)

Ironically, a few months later we arrived on the wards to find the Southampton footballers split into groups and on each of the wards – and I thought of that quote. I knew immediately they were there as I could smell the heady mix of many different aftershaves lingering in the corridors. It's funny because they were in identical kit but they certainly didn't align their fragrances! Leo looked most put out that he wasn't the centre of attention that day as everyone was requesting a selfie or an autograph and it didn't help that some of the players were, initially anyway, terrified of dogs. But it was OK because the players who were dog lovers showed that the therapy dogs were something special – after all, they were interacting with children – and Leo was no threat to them whatsoever.

In no time at all everyone was wanting selfies with Leo and a plan was hatched to have a group photo with the dog. The official photographer stepped back to take the picture of the players resplendent in their white tracksuits. Leo, sitting in the middle of them watching me, suddenly started to twitch his nose. I looked over, raised my hand above the photographer's shoulder to get the dog to look at me and ... aaatttiiiisshoooo! Leo sneezed the biggest sneeze I've ever heard! The mix of aftershave got to him and everyone fell about laughing.

As things settled at home with our new girl, Pollyanna, our minds turned to our eldest son Harry's Master's degree graduation ceremony, which was taking place at the Albert Hall in London. It was a fantastic day and of course once the ceremony was over and we were back outside I wanted to take as many photographs as possible of him in his gown. In the middle of it all, I took a call from the Kennel Club to say that Leo and I were finalists in the their 'Friends for Life' competition, 2020, but, we could not tell a soul! Even on that special day the dogs somehow managed to find their way into family life.

Knowing that Donna and the paediatric intensive care team were responsible for our successful nomination for the 'Child's Champion' category was just amazing. I was familiar with the competition, so I knew that the winners in each category are decided by public vote ahead of *Crufts*, but to know that our healthcare professional peers had put Leo and I (well, as I see it, the entire team really: Karen, Hannah and Liz and all the other dogs on the team, too) forward for the award was really special to me. I felt proud of my main man Leo and pleased that he would be beside me in the main ring when the winner would be announced, and of course I really wanted that to be – Lyndsey and Leo! I wanted it for the clinical team at the hospital and for our therapy dog team because the past year had seen so much development and even more acceptance for the therapy dog team at SCH.

I reminded myself again that, somehow, we had visited over 2,500 patients in twelve months, both in the hospital and those receiving palliative care at home and in the hospice. It was quite an achievement thinking that we did it through weekday, weekend, holiday and half-term visits, special activities, and ad hoc and home visits; there was so much to do and the more there was, the more we did. But luck has been with me from day one and the determination to keep doing the one thing I've really felt a calling to do – especially with Leo at my side.

The nomination made me think about the people who had opened doors for me because of their belief in the therapy dogs. I remember Professor Clarke giving us his full support and welcoming us onto his paediatric orthopaedic ward – even before Mike did! But then, he had seen therapy dogs benefiting patients in the USA and understood completely. It was fate that led to a conversation with Marla at Denver University. Up until that conversation I had convinced myself that I didn't have the qualifications to take their Animals and Human Health course in Animal Assisted Intervention. That course, the people and the experience fired me up and set my mind racing, thinking about the scope of what our therapy dogs could offer the clinical staff and the patients, as they do in some specialist places across the world. From the moment I gained my qualification I was like a dog with a bone!

As we sped towards the end of 2019, I had begun to get my head around some of the other reasons why we had been nominated for the 'Friends for Life' award and my thoughts drifted back to other ideas that had been put into effect over the previous few years. Preparation and planning were a big part of the learning on my course and while our team usually has a dog on the wards at some point four to five days a week, I wanted to be able to provide support when we couldn't be present. That's where the pre-op test pictures and YouTube videos appeared.

In the summer of 2017, with Ollie soon off to university to study film and French, I had drafted him in to film *Leo Goes to X-ray* and he soon came up with a creative idea to show that there's no need to be scared of the large complicated technical equipment in radiology, including the huge cumbersome scanners that you go through. The next one, filmed a couple of years later during his university summer holiday, *Leo Goes to Theatre*, captured Leo taking the route from the ward to theatre, taking the same steps that the children take – to show that if Leo can do it, it's not scary at all. Suddenly we had a hit on our hands, as proven in August 2020 when a mum shared that after watching the video, her daughter, little two-year-old Millie, said: 'Just like Leo' as the anaesthetist put the mask over her face!

Leo was also requested to model by the paediatric cardiology team, but I felt that it might be too risky asking him to lie on his back for an ultrasound scan of his chest – we just might see more than we wanted! So, Jessie was brought in and she lay so beautifully still with me holding her paw. We took lots of photographs which I shared on Twitter. At the time, as a rookie Twitter user, I had previously set the dogs up using Jessie's date of birth. All seemed to go fine, but soon after we joined we were banned for a week for being underage! Once I had revised the details all seemed to be ticking along just fine until the images of Jessie's belly were picked up by @dog_rates who gave her 14/10 for being a good doggo and shared thousands of times in a few hours – @schtherapydogs was banned for another week as the Twitter algorithms clearly weren't too sure about us. All we could do was watch as Jessie's belly went viral! The world and its grandma wanted to know what we were doing – even Yahoo! Australia wrote a piece about us!

It was all a very exciting whirlwind, as was the arrival in November of the film crew from the Kennel Club to capture some footage of Leo and the team doing their duty on the wards, in advance of *Crufts* 2020 in March. I wondered if some of the parents would be happy to take part, as not everyone is OK with having this sensitive part of their life committed to film.

I was so pleased that we could share the story of baby George Lowther who was just six days old when he was rushed into the emergency department with suspected meningitis. Later, doctors discovered that his heart was failing due to myocarditis and so began the little one's four-month stay in hospital. It wasn't just George's parents, Adam and Emily, who loved to see the dogs and enjoy Leo's company as a piece of escape back to normality: George's three-year-old brother, Theo, looked forward to cuddling Leo too. Sometimes it was being able to see Leo that made the short visits to see his baby brother bearable after his life was turned upside down. To be able to hug, laugh and sometimes cry with Leo was just what this family, and others, needed.

I was also pleased when Oscar's parents said they would take part. Oscar, the boy who smiled for the first time on meeting Leo, was going to be part of 'Friends for Life' too. Since that day, Leo and all the other therapy dogs had played a part in Oscar's treatment programme, which involved physiotherapy, occupational and speech therapy. We made Playdough paws and painted pictures with Leo in support of this, and Jessie also assisted in Oscar's physiotherapy sessions in an Animal Assisted Therapy mini-version of the game 'pass the box of dog biscuits'. Lifting the box passed to him by his brother, Ollie, turning towards his physio and finally ... Jessie, who gratefully received the delicious-smelling booty. Needless to say, we did it a few times before the box was opened and her tail wagged like crazy.

Leo later supported Oscar through an MRI scan – by then the little boy was aged six – which he did without sedation after watching our *Leo Goes to X-ray* video. Using the intercom during the procedure, the radiographer let him know that Leo was still waiting for him and would be there when he finished. Oscar lay still for the twenty-two minutes of the scan. I'd wondered if it would work – but it did and he was so relieved to see Leo waiting for him when it was all over and he was out of the huge machine. Leo's magical presence worked for Ollie, Oscar's brother, too. Leo was there to support Ollie during the first part of Oscar's illness. We chatted to him and painted pictures that he could take into school with lots of Leo stickers for his classmates. It was something else for him to talk about when he made it into the classroom that wasn't to do with his poorly sibling. Our version of AAI at SCH and Leo, in all his golden goodness, had so much to offer these children.

When I was invited to visit Oscar's school with Leo to hold an assembly for his year group, we took Leo cards and a bunch of stickers to give out – the children love them – and, for once, it put Oscar at the centre of the action. At age seven, he was finding the return to school tough and we thought taking Leo in would be a great icebreaker with his classmates. Before we went in, of course, the school had written to the parents of children who were involved to check for allergies or if anyone preferred that their child didn't encounter the dog for any reason. Staff also asked parents to send in any pictures of their children with SCH therapy dogs, if they have ever seen them doing their rounds.

The school visit was near Bognor Regis, over forty miles away from Southampton, so only patients transferred to a specialist centre would be there. Consequently, when I asked if anyone had a picture that included the dogs, I didn't expect what happened next. Four children put their hands up. Oscar and two other boys had pictures of themselves with Leo or one of his friends, so I asked them to come and sit with me. And then a girl put her hand up and showed me a picture of her sister, who we saw before she died. She joined me too, getting right up close to cuddle Leo, and stayed cuddling him the whole time I was there. Shocking to me was the realisation that four in that small year-group assembly had either been patients at SCH or a sibling of a patient in what seemed such a short time since we started our therapy dog service. I then had four children sitting with me at the front, Leo first sitting beside the children with me and then as he got a little bit more tired, he lay down, ending up lying with his head in the lap of the bereaved girl.

The *Friends for Life* pre-filming in the can, it was good to get back to normal visits within the hospital and then just look forward to the big day in March. We were also able to embark on a study of the physiological benefits of our visits to patients in PICU as, incredibly, the all-important ethics approval for the study had been granted. The difficulty was keeping the news that we were competition finalists quiet for so many weeks! The families involved in the *Friends for Life* film had been sworn to secrecy and everyone else around the hospital too. It was such an honour to be nominated by our peers and I wanted to make sure that the nomination reflected a team effort with fellow handlers Karen, Hannah and Liz beside me, and Jessie, Quinn, Archie, Hattie and Milo at our feet. I could not have achieved this on my own. And as I write this, I stroke Leo at the same time because he was with me in those early days, taking over as Monty retired. I think of the journey, the people and how their stories illuminate the scope of a therapy dog's ability to assist.

I think of a patient we were asked to visit in adult intensive care by Dr Max Jonas. The patient, Billy, lived on the streets of Southampton with his dog at his side and his admission to hospital meant that they had been separated for the first time since they met. Billy was gravely ill and missing his dog so much that it took just stroking Leo to bring him great comfort as he faced an uncertain future.

I think of the time a police investigation team were on PICU and they had been there for seventy-two hours with limited rest. I remember walking onto the ward and checking in with Donna to see a specific patient and ask if there was anyone else who might be on the list for our meet-and-greet. As we left after our visit a police officer came over from a different part of the ward and asked if she could stroke Leo. She crouched on the floor with a very nudgy dog for several minutes before getting back on her feet and saying that it was the best moment in the past few days and how wonderful it was to see a dog on the ward. It allowed the officer to switch off from the environment, her work, her stress and to just relax. I was deeply touched by these words. To be able to do that is exactly why I do what I do with my dogs.

And, it seems, we do it even if we are not 'on duty', as happened with Lewis Parfoot, who was in his early twenties and being treated for non-Hodgkin's lymphoma when he saw Leo and I walking across the hospital car park and headed straight for us. Every arranged visit to Lewis after that helped with the emotional stress of his cancer treatment, every second spent with Leo inspired him to smile again – and, with all the support of his girlfriend, Sophie – to have a golden retriever of their own.

This is what I want to give to the families – comfort and distraction, to allow them space and time to not be a patient or the parent of a critically ill child. To give children like the Curtis brothers, Harry and Josh, who each faced a daunting time in hospital and surgery, the company of a cuddly, canine companion to ease their fears. And a photograph of their super-hero, Leo, to remind them of their courage. Stroking Leo gave comfort and shed light and warmth on a scary situation. Stroking him put hope into the moment. And hope is what carries us through life, no matter how old we are.

32

'If I give something back …'

I STILL FEEL INDEBTED TO THE HOSPITAL that gave Ollie back his health and his future, but in many ways, it has also given me so much too: a sense of worth, some great times, some sad times and so many times where I find myself feeling rebalanced after visiting with my therapy dogs. It is truly a place where some great people work, some fabulous strangers are met and memories created. All of us on the team have called SCH our happy place at different times. Together we have shared tears of relief, sadness and frustration. I know that I will shed many, many more as we take what we have achieved and build on it to reach more children, more families in this special way. We have only just started out on a road that is stretched out in front of us – with dogs as our partners in every way.

For me, the role of a therapy dog represents the epitome of the human-animal bond. There is something so inexplicable about it that you really have to experience it to believe in it. One thing is for sure: it is a very powerful connection that exists only to do good in this world. We are so fortunate that dogs want to key into our vulnerability and build us up to be the best versions of ourselves. They never set out to weaken or criticise or punish us for being imperfect, because they love us just the way we are. I know when I accepted the Kennel Club 'Friends for Life' winner's trophy, Leo was beside me physically, emotionally and, yes, in my psyche. He is my partner in care, the yin to my yang and the dog who has taught me the absolute power of kindness.

Thank you, Leo. You are my flump, an old soul who just knows about people and what they need to make them feel better. Isn't it true, if you love them, somehow dogs can make everything better at the worst of times?

Epilogue

I'M SOMETIMES ASKED IF LEO IS MY FAVOURITE. At the hospital I have to confess that he is my favourite partner for AAI as he is so in tune with the role and he has a special, knowing connection with children.

It is probably not right to consider favourites, though. Each of my dogs has been my favourite for one reason or another, as their individual personalities have merged into and enhanced our family. Truth is, I love them all for being exactly who they are: Monty for his solid loyalty and silent wisdom when I was experiencing dark thoughts; Totty for being my perfect earthmother with her pups and my brilliant running partner; Jessie for her big jolly personality; Quinn the perfect blend of handsome Leo and smiley Jessie; Pollyanna for being my beautiful clever girl; and Leo for just being Leo and instinctively knowing when I need him most. They are all special and their gift to me has been their willingness to be my partners in my mission to take all aspects of Animal Assisted Intervention onto hospital wards. Let's face it, I would have been lost without them. Despite being the same breed, they are all different and I love them for their individual characteristics. I am often asked why the girls do less than the boys and it is simply the fact that they take quite a while off when they are in season, so have less opportunity to build their experience week after week. Nevertheless, they are still great at what they do, are very much a part of the team and always will be.

Sometimes you should never look back but just be thankful that you made it through whatever phase of life you are in. When I was first approached to write a book, it took me a while to agree, but slowly, as the Covid-19 lockdown continued, it all seemed to fall into place. I was persuaded that there are times when you must glance over your shoulder to appreciate how you survived the journey and negotiated the bumps in the road. I admit that I'm not sure where I would be in this life had it not evolved into one shared with dogs. When our young son, Ollie, was diagnosed with acute myeloid leukaemia, my old life crashed to a halt. But then, three years later, his all-clear put my life on an unexpected and amazing trajectory. I had hope and a deal I had made with myself to deliver. Our family had survived the worst of times and there to help were the dogs, and not for the first time. I owe them so much and I always will.

Sharing Leo & friends as therapy dogs with other parents and children remains a huge privilege. I could choose to reflect on our role in the patients' sometimes difficult healthcare journeys, but instead I remember them and their families finding joy and peace in sharing the best of the human-animal bond – and smiling. We stay in contact with many of the families of the multitude of children we have supported, including those we call our 'angel' patients. This book tells of just a few, but as a team we have seen over 10,000 patients since I first started in 2012; I could not have imagined the Pandora's box I was opening in my life but I am so glad I did. There is no 'I' in team though and we would not have come so far had I not been joined by Karen, Hannah and Liz with their golden retrievers, who were all reared by me. I am a lucky lady to have been given the opportunity to create this team with good friends and a family of dogs I know so well.

Sadly, I could not include all of the stories I wanted to in these pages and I'm sure that as soon as I stop typing, I will recall a thousand more that I want to add to *Leo & Friends*, but we have to close somewhere. What I want to share with you is that I am grateful for the opportunity to be invited into the lives of families in their difficult times and to be able to offer our version of Animal Assisted Intervention. And I am so grateful to the healthcare professionals at Southampton Children's Hospital, part of University Hospital Southampton NHS Trust, for their foresight. Some of our patients have been seen briefly on the day ward while others have been inpatients for something much more complex that required a longer stay. We have seen them on all of the wards and supported patients through surgery, rehabilitation and long-term recovery. It doesn't matter to us why they are in hospital, if we have been on the wards and they've wanted to share a little bit of canine magic it has been our pleasure to do so.

Our rewards are the smiles and the pleasure it gives us. There are so many photographs with the dogs captured in treasured snapshots and keepsakes. There are also many memories of times when my 'hobby' probably supports the 'crazy dog lady' title. Who suggested we get permission to go with seven dogs into John Lewis, Southampton to take photographs for an advent calendar for Christmas 2019? Yes, me!

During the Covid-19 pandemic we had to suspend our visits to the hospital and that was one of the hardest things I have ever had to accept. As a team we were disappointed. On a personal level I felt empty and at a loss to know what to do as I watched our professional colleagues burdened with the overwhelming task of providing healthcare in a pandemic. I had tears in my eyes as I removed our visiting kit from my car when, after a few weeks of lockdown, it became apparent we would be off for a long time.

We filled the gap for the patients as best we could, with 'Dogtor Leo' and the rest of the crew giving briefings on social media and YouTube. I learned to use some basic film-editing software and we filmed the dogs doing all sorts of things – out on their walks getting dirty, showering and having a grooming 'makeover', having a story read to them, lockdown baking and other crazy things just to entertain the children that we couldn't go in to see. We also saw some of the patients on Zoom visits and enjoyed catching up with them, albeit remotely.

So where does the future lie? When I started in 2012, few in the UK had heard of Animal Assisted Intervention in healthcare, yet now it can be found being presented at national and international conferences alongside some of the more traditional medical scientific advances. Our SCH

Therapy Dogs team became full members of Animal Assisted Intervention International in 2020. It is wonderful to see their board developing an international set of standards which is being continually enhanced to help ensure the future progression of AAI in a safe way, for both the animals and the humans involved in the partnership.

As far as UK healthcare is concerned, Kate Tantam's talk to the 8th Annual Critical Care Rehabilitation Conference in Baltimore, USA, entitled 'Morale with a Tail', opened up more discussion on the use of AAI in critical care. Her #rehablegend idea is that intensive care rehabilitation is of huge benefit to patients in the long term ... and that can include working with a therapy dog too. Our new study with Dr Michael Griksaitis and advanced nurse practitioner Donna Austin in Southampton Children's Hospital paediatric intensive care unit is researching the physiological benefits of AAI and this will continue as soon as we return to 'work'. We look forward to seeing what results that will bring.

As I finalise writing this, we are in the early days of the lockdown being lifted in England in 2021 and I can't wait to put my AAI kit back into the car and get the dogs ready to go back to their ward duties! I will take each dog individually for shorter visits for the first few weeks to make sure they have still 'got it'. I hope the whole team will return successfully, but they are dogs and if one or more indicates they are no longer comfortable then so be it. They are our pets first and foremost.

When Nick Brooks-Ward, the arena director and commentator at *Crufts*, spoke to me after our win in the

'Friends for Life' competition in 2020, he told me how delighted he was. It turned out we had supported one of his family members while they were in intensive care. I *knew* I recognised him when he introduced us in the ring! We talked and he said: 'The thing about dogs is if we look after them, they will look after us.' How right he was and it is my duty to look after my pack. When we return to work, I feel sure each of them will show me what their decision is, although I have a feeling I know who will look at me as if to say ... 'Right, I'm back, now where are my patients?'

I know that dogs have the power to support patients through their hospitalisation and healing process as long as there are no contraindications to them being near dogs. I see it happen with our therapy dog family every time we walk the wards of the hospital. Where Monty, Totty and Jessie started, Leo has healed me too and I am grateful for his help in finding my way to a fulfilling role helping others. I believe that Leo and I were put on this path together and am so glad Catherine chose him for me.

We cannot fix anyone, that is down to the healthcare professionals, but we can break down the barriers presented by a clinical environment and give the patients something good and familiar to trust in. Our role is to make positive memories and the dogs are a little bit of magic to cling to in a storm.

In my book, that has to be a gift worth sharing.

Roll call

THE DOGS HAVE BEEN PERFORMING their special canine magic at Southampton Children's Hospital since 2012 alongside a cast of more than 10,000 patients. It would be impossible to name everyone, but I hold memories of all those with whom my dogs have spent time enjoying the human-animal bond. Some brief memories follow below ... all of them are cherished.

Many of these patients you have already met within the pages of the book and I am grateful to the parents and children who gave their testimonies and contributions so generously so that the reader could understand the impact of our visits. A very big thank you to you all. All of these memories helped give me the extra nudge to agree to write the book. The list below is in no particular order but written as it flowed ...

ALICE – the girl who secured Monty's place at the top of our canine roll call when he persuaded you out of your room for the first time.

ROSINA – because I will never forget the birthday cake 'incident' and rushing down to M&S for the new one!

BARRY – for showing us that the magic of Animal Assisted Intervention works with adults sedated in intensive care too.

FELIX – I will never forget your incredible walk outside with Leo and the physiotherapy team. Your athlete's mindset certainly showed in the distance you covered.

ARCHIE – whose vital signs improved and the first tweet went out about AAI in the paediatric intensive care unit at SCH.

DYLAN – for the time you went on your special trip to *Crufts* and giving away our secrets on BBC *South Today*!

LIBBY – who despite her sedation making her feel sleepy in intensive care still managed a beautiful smile when she saw Leo.

GEORGE – the baby who went from life under a mask in PICU to the little chap with the biggest smile.

JO – the girl who I just had to make a home visit happen for so she could have puppy therapy when Jessie had her litter.

LEWIS – for being the special little boy that you are, who loved to reach out and feel Leo and now has his own special dog.

GRACIE – the media star alongside Hattie and the girl who loved to introduce the new children to the therapy dogs during her treatment.

OSCAR – whose smile for Leo gave his family hope as they waited to see what would happen during his time in intensive care.

BEN – who loved Lego, *The Avengers*, *Guardians of the Galaxy* and golden retriever visits!

JAMES – for all the times when the dogs made you smile and all your incredible Lego creativity.

ELLIE – whose incredible artwork of the dogs is a gift we can all still enjoy.

BECCA – who was in for ages and said: 'Therapy dogs were a girl's best friend, not diamonds.'

JOAN – your bony hand in mine lingered and I knew our visit meant the world to you.

GEORGE – who has three of his own golden retrievers but still thinks Leo is his special hospital friend.

TORRI – who loved our virtual visit on Zoom so she could see where the dogs lived, what they get up to at home and see all of them at the same time!

EMILY – for having her special box of dog treats with her at all times visiting you and Pollyanna on her first home visit.

SHEYLAN – who showed that despite being non-verbal and with little understanding of English, the language of the human-animal bond spoke to you.

EMILY – for a special time when we waited with you to go to theatre and you shared Leo with a boy who said he was scared of dogs.

FINLEY – who was scared at first as he didn't like dogs but decided he could trust Leo. By the end of our visit, he was brushing and stroking Leo *and* feeding him treats!

SOPHIE – whose favourite animal is her cat but enjoyed seeing the therapy dogs, who found her wind-up tweety bird very curious.

LILLIAN – because both you and Leo learned how to wear an anaesthetic mask in the same week!

GEORGE – sometimes a fireman, policeman, ambulance driver, army officer, pirate ... a boy with all the costumes – and one huge dog lover, just like his sister, Bella.

HARRY – who has a picture of Leo in his bedroom and says: 'When I feel scared about hospital I think of Leo and then I feel OK.'

CLOÉ – whose mother wrote to thank the PICU team as well as 'Leo (le chien) et sa maîtresse'.

ZOÉ – the Princess. Lover of ladybirds, dogs and all things in nature.

LOTTIE – who we met numerous times on the wards and now has her own assistance dog that helps her so much.

JAKE – who had just come out of a coma and started talking about his dog at home.

LEWIS – now four years in remission. Aged 25 during treatment, he was missing his new puppy Humphrey at home, so had some huge Leo cuddles the day before he went into isolation for his stem cell transplant.

CONNIE – for the smiles and teenage chats whenever you have been in.

MILLIE – who is now 19 but loved meeting Leo in PICU the day before she went to London for a lung transplant five years ago.

CHARLIE – and her sister Emmy, who told me all about their golden retriever, Maisie, when Charlie was in for an operation.

DANIEL – for all the times the dogs supported you and helped you get to theatre ... And of course for their sausage salaries!

MAUREEN – for the kind words you said about the difference we make when working with Claire and her colleagues.

TATE – because even if you are in isolation you can still high-five a dog through the window!

KATIE – who always reminded us that Archie and Leo were actually 'her boys'.

ANNIE – whose consultant arranged for us to escort her into the anaesthetic room and it made all the difference.

GEORGIA – who uses Makaton to talk but could always get the dogs to know what she was saying.

KEIRA – for being a star in our special Christmas video, where the dogs were the 'elves'!

MILLIE – aged two, who watched *Leo Goes to Theatre* before her admission and when she saw the anaesthetic mask said: 'like Leo', despite us not being able to be there because of the Covid lockdown.

ROISIN – for those big hugs you had, the special pictures with Quinn and how you are now inspiring others.

NOAH – for the times when you just couldn't resist holding the dogs close for longer.

EDITH – for ringing the end-of-treatment bell at home with your sister Eleanor and your surprise when the dogs popped round.

BECKY – who says Leo was her 'first dog' and went on to recover and join the nursing profession.

BROOKE – who loved Leo, especially when, wearing a 'lion's mane', he turned up in her living room.

NIXON – who learnt to sign 'Leo' before any other word.

YASMIN – who shared a special time on the ward with Milo, who enjoyed all the fuss.

BILLY – who told Leo how he worried about his friends looking after his dog on the streets.

LIVVY – for our verse in your beautiful poem:

Chemo means I've met nice people
I would never have met before.
The nurses and doctors are kind and caring
And I love it when Leo appears at my door.

... and literally thousands more.

Some of the patients we've seen are babies who've grown into school children, some are now adults and, sadly, some are angels, but we think of you all and will always treasure the memories of time spent with you. Leo and friends send big fluffy hugs, as always.

It is our privilege to have spent time with you.

Acknowledgements

AS I'VE SAID BEFORE, there is no 'I' in team and I am certain that I would not be where I am today without Leo and a whole host of others. Monty, Totty and Jessie, Leo's canine predecessors, introduced me to home life with golden retrievers and ultimately to volunteering as a Pets As Therapy handler, which led me into the world of Animal Assisted Intervention.

I need to acknowledge so many who have contributed to this book, directly or indirectly.

My human family, and most especially Mike, Harry and Ollie. Friends, both human and canine! Huge thanks must also go to the professional staff at Southampton Children's Hospital who've allowed me to develop the team and of course the team itself, both dogs and handlers. Without Karen, Hannah, Liz and all of our canine colleagues we would never have developed such a service at the hospital.

I also need to thank my ghost-writer, Isabel George, who took the tens of thousands of words that I'd written and created what you see here – believe me, reader, you should be grateful too! If it had been left to me this would be an enormous ring binder of lists, Post-it notes, phone-recorded brain dumps, emails, Word documents and very, very long paragraphs!

Thanks must also go to Kelly Ellis, publishing director, and editor Holly Blood at HarperCollins as well as Kate Latham and our agent Clare Hulton, who expertly guided me through the whole process.

This book has many contributors and of course the most important ones I need to thank are the thousands of patients and families who've allowed us to be with them on whatever healthcare path they were taking. I have met some incredible people and made some very special memories. This book is a testimony to the power of the human-animal bond in healthcare and we are grateful to them for allowing our dogs to share it via AAI at Southampton Children's Hospital and University Hospital Southampton NHS Trust.

Other contributors who gave both time and details for the book and therefore deserve special mention in no particular order:

Amanda Cheesley, formerly Professional Lead for Long Term Conditions and End of Life Care, Royal College of Nursing, now Chair of Sirona Care & Health CIC

Dr Amy Savage, Clinical Psychologist, Southampton Children's Hospital

Donna Austin, Advanced Nurse Practitioner, Paediatric Intensive Care Unit, Southampton Children's Hospital

Jan Tait, Children's Orthopaedic Nurse Practitioner, Southampton Children's Hospital

Joyce Stebbings, Youth and Play Service Manager, Southampton Children's Hospital

June Gallagher, Senior Sister, Southampton Children's Hospital

Kate Gatehouse, Paediatric Physiotherapist, Southampton Children's Hospital

Kate Pye, former Divisional Head of Nursing, Southampton Children's Hospital (now Head of Nursing, Paediatric Cancer, Great Ormond Street Hospital)

Kate Tantam, Specialist Senior Sister, Intensive Care Rehabilitation Team, Plymouth Hospitals NHS Trust

Dr Michael Griksaitis, Consultant, Paediatric Intensive Care Unit, Southampton Children's Hospital

Dr Max Jonas, Consultant, General Intensive Care Unit, Southampton University Hospital NHS Trust

Prof. Nicholas Clarke, Consultant Paediatric Orthopaedic Surgeon, Southampton Children's Hospital (now retired)

The above are (or were) staff at University Hospital Southampton NHS Trust and others that I contacted when researching for this book. There are many more that we have worked alongside since 2012 and without whom our Animal Assisted Intervention would never have got this far. They have welcomed our 'pack' across the hospital and I am grateful to them all for allowing us to create what we are proud to share with the patients and their families.

I also owe a huge debt of thanks to the following, again in no particular order:

Catherine and Sven Zingg of Rayleas Golden Retrievers, who gave me details of Sarah, who had used one of their stud dogs when I wanted my first dog – the rest is history! Their continued support and interest in what we do is invaluable.

Sarah and Patrick Curry, who made my thirty-five-year dream of owning a golden retriever come true with Monty and then later with Totty.

Alexandra Butler, our vet, who is always there for all of us, canine and human, when we are worried!

Professor Noel Fitzpatrick and his team for treating Leo after his accident.

Fitzpatrick Referrals for their kind permission to film Leo in their scanner for the *Leo Goes to X-ray* video when it was proving impossible to find hospital scanners without patients in them!

Pets As Therapy – the UK charity I first registered with in 2012 and very soon had the most incredible hobby!

Daniel Howarth Illustration for the 'Leo with the stethoscope' logo and other pictures for the children.

… and also those educators, mentors and other professionals that I have been in contact with over the last few years as things have been developing:

Professor Phil Tedeschi and his team at the Institute for Human Animal Connection, University of Denver, especially Marla who encouraged me so much when I enquired.

Ann Howie, Human-Animal Solutions, mentor and author of *Teaming with Your Therapy Dog* and *The Handler Factor*.

Dr Aubrey Fine, mentor and author of the *Handbook on Animal Assisted Therapy*.

The Humanimal Trust for their support for our study: 'The Benefits of an Animal Assisted Intervention service to patients and staff at a children's hospital', published in the *British Journal of Nursing*, April 2019.

The Royal College of Nursing 'Working with Dogs in Health Care Settings' committee members, who I worked with to create the national guidelines for healthcare facilities. First published May 2018, with revision and addendum for high-risk areas December 2019.

The Intensive Care Society committee I sat on to create the 'Guidance for Animal Assisted Intervention (AAI) in a Critical Care Setting', October 2020.

Animal Assisted Intervention International for recognising Southampton Children's Hospital therapy dog team as full members since 2020.

Finally, I must again thank my handler colleagues and friends Karen, Liz and Hannah. Without you joining me, we would never have come so far. One woman and one dog could never have seen more than ten thousand patients and

I am grateful to you for sharing the passion for the visits and, of course, your friendship. Behind the scenes we spend hours discussing things and planning to ensure the patients and staff receive the best support from the right handler and dog team. That can only be done with colleagues who are friends and dogs who can work well together.

I feel very honoured to be here with Leo as the Kennel Club of Great Britain, 'Friends for Life' Champion 2020, but it has to be considered a team accolade ... We do it because we are Leo & Friends.